i

NO Antibiotics... NO Side Effects...
NO Controversy... NO Politics!

Biting Back

How to Naturally Overcome the Chronic Effects of Lyme Disease and Other Tick-Triggered Illness... After All Else Has Failed

Donald K. Liebell, D.C., B.C.A.O.

Foreword by Nader Soliman, M.D.
Edited by Donna Zampi, Ph.D. and Laura Veach, Ph.D.

Copyright 2015 by Donald K. Liebell, DC, BCAO (Updated 2018)
Published and Printed in the United States of America by
CreateSpace Independent Publishing Platform, North Charleston, SC

ISBN-13: 978-1511731577   ISBN-10: 1511731575
Library of Congress Control Number: 2015912462

Publisher's Note

Dedication

To my best friend and love of my life, my wife, Sheila Liebell, whose perseverance, strength, intelligence, and support made Biting Back possible. Because of her experience, perseverance, and strength, I have been able to pursue the knowledge and skill to guide victims of this dreadful disease back to a state of health.

To my beloved mother, Barbara Liebell, who raised me with natural health principles, and pointed me towards the path I have followed—long before holistic wellness became popular or in public demand. She didn't need a doctoral degree to teach me that the human body can heal itself, and that true health is natural health.

To my mentor in acupuncture and homeopathy, Dr. Nader Soliman, who took the drastically under-utilized works of scientific geniuses... made them even *better*... and personally taught me how to replicate those skills, enabling me to consistently help restore sick and suffering people's health and quality of life—without a single drug!

Preface and Disclaimer

The concept of free speech has its limitations. It also has its risks. I wish it were not necessary to write this preface and disclaimer, but here goes: Everything you read in Biting Back is based upon my personal experience and research into a number of health topics, and it is for educational purposes only.

I am making no attempt to instruct readers to self-diagnose or treat any medical condition. Nor am I suggesting discontinuation of the services of any doctor or therapist, or any medical treatment. Any commentary on long-term antibiotic usage is for general information purposes only. I am licensed by the Virginia Board of Medicine in both chiropractic and acupuncture. Thus, I do not prescribe medication, nor do I ever advise patients on either its use or disuse, both in print or verbally.

Biting Back presents *my* natural, wellness-based, whole-body approach to treatment. It is not portrayed as a replacement for, or delay for undergoing any conventional medical evaluation or treatment. It is a treatment option, which may be used in conjunction with any other medical treatment, or as a sole approach, at my patients' discretion. By definition, the practice of medicine has always included any and all means by which human health may be improved. I believe nobody should ever feel torn between conventional pharmaceutical-based medicine and natural holistic approaches. They each have their role, and in an effective medical system, should be complementary and compatible, but never antagonistic. I repeat that this book is for educational awareness purposes only, and the reader is solely responsible for his or her own health care choices.

Donald Liebell, DC, BCAO
Chronic Pain & Wellness Solutions
www.Hope4Lyme.com   www.LiebellClinic.com

Contents

Foreword by Nader Soliman, MD
Introduction

Part One: Crushing the Controversies and Conundrums

Chapter 1: How a Frazzled Mother-of-Three, Desperate for Answers and Losing Hope… *Conquered* Chronic Lyme Disease (In a Matter of Months)… <u>Without</u> Antibiotics, Other Drugs, Herbs, or Complicated Diets (Page 16)

Chapter 2: If You are Losing the Battle, Switch the Battlefield! How to Avoid "Lyme Wars," Risky Treatments, Controversial Tests, and Improve Your Physical and Mental Health (Page 20)

Part Two: Debunking Diagnosis Disasters

Chapter 3: Borrelia Band Blunders & the Dangerous Delusion of Diagnosis (Page 27)

Chapter 4: Why Conventional Western Medicine is a <u>Lemon</u> for Lyme (Page 31)

Chapter 5: The Diagnosis You Dread… *"It's All in Your Head!"* (Page 46)

Chapter 6: Metallic Misdiagnosis Mayhem: The Toxic Substances Your Body Can't Properly Purge Out (Some People Spend Thousands of Dollars Trying To Eliminate It—Not Realizing Why It Will Keep Coming Back) (Page 51)

Chapter 7: Microbes without Medicine: The "Dirty Little Secret" that Keeps Victims of Tick-Borne Illness Sick (Page 56)

Chapter 8: Adrenal Fatigue: How Can a Medical Problem So Serious Get So Little Attention? (Page 65)

Part Three: Myths, Misconceptions, and Mistakes— What NOT to Do (and Why)

Chapter 9: Drug Obsessions and Prescription Confessions— Why Antibiotics May Not Be the Answer (Page 71)

Chapter 10: The Detoxification Abomination: Why You Must Not Forcefully "Detox" (Most Methods Out There Are Disastrous, Painful, Unhealthy, And Simply *Wrong!*) (Page 89)

Chapter 11: Sleep Cycle Sadness and Melatonin Madness: Learn Why a Good Night's Sleep Requires More than a Prescription or Melatonin Supplements (Page 93)

Chapter 12: Treatment with Rife? Not on Your Life! Why Rife Machines Should Be Avoided. Even If These Frequency Generators Really *Do* Kill Lyme *Borrelia* Bacteria... They Are *Not* What They're Cracked Up To Be! (Page 100)

Chapter 13: Glutathione Gluttony and Glorification? Do You *Really* Need to Obsess Over This Antioxidant to Get Better? (Page 103)

Chapter 14: Taking The Rut Out Of "Leaky Gut:" Discover Why You May Be Flushing Money Down The Drain With Supplements... And What You Can Do To Ensure Great Nutrition And Nutrient Absorption   (Page 105)

Chapter 15: Why Herbal Medicine Is Likely *Not* The Answer (Hint: Herbs Fail For The *Same* Reason As When Antibiotics Fail!) (Page 113)

Chapter 16: The "More is Better" Betrayal: Why Simplifying Your Approach Leads to a Better Outcome (Page 116)

Chapter 17: Who Are The True Health Authorities? (Page 118)

Part Four: The Bio-energetic Individual Treatment Equation

Chapter 18: Immune System 101: A Simple Explanation of Your Body's Inborn Defense System, and Why it is Capable of Overcoming Lyme Disease and Many Other Illnesses (Page 132)

Chapter 19: The Subtle Signals of Bio-electric Fields: How a Resurrected "Pearl Of Wisdom" From a Yale Anatomy Professor's Research Provides Health Clues That Blood Tests <u>Miss</u>! (Page 142)

Chapter 20: Look to the Auricle: How a French Neurologist's Strange Discovery About The Human *Ear* In 1957 Could Be Part of Your Chronic Lyme Disease Solution Today (It's Endorsed by the *World Health Organization*, and Published in Medical Journals, But It's Rarely Practiced *Correctly* In The U.S.) (Page 150)

Chapter 21: An Earful of Wisdom: How the Ear is Used to Determine Treatment Needs… and Why it Does NOT Matter Whether or Not You Have Been "Officially" Diagnosed With Lyme Disease (Page 157)

Chapter 22: Clearing Energetic Blockages of the Brain: The First Step Towards Recovery…The Little-Known, Neurological Problem That Must Be Detected and Treated to Ensure Successful Treatment (Page 173)

Chapter 23: Patient-Centered Holistic Wellness (Page 180)

Chapter 24: Homeopathic Principles to the Rescue (Page 182)

Chapter 25: Bio-energetic Wellness Support Supplementation—the Breakthrough Modern Homeopathic Wellness Technology That Could Be the Key to Your Recovery (Page 194)

Chapter 26: The Weakest Link—Why Neck Health is a Critical Part of the Equation (Page 216)

Chapter 27: D Deficiency Dilemma: What Nobody Has Told You About Vitamin D Supplements   (Page 235)

Chapter 28: Fantastic Food Fortification: Why Superior Nutrition Through Whole Foods Trumps Taking Expensive, Processed Vitamin and Mineral Supplements (Page 238)

Chapter 29: Navigating the Road to Wellness (Page 241)

Part Five: Diffusing the Doubters, Detractors, and Disparagers

Chapter 30: Discernment: Who Are The Kooks And Charlatans? (Page 247)

Chapter 31: Putting Placebo Proclaimers in Their Place: Why Cries of Placebo Effect Do Not Hold Water (Page 261)

Chapter 32: Why Some People Respond to Treatment Better Than Others (Page 275)

Chapter 33: "Evidence-Based Medicine" Evil—Why This Proposed New Standard for Practicing Medicine Tragically Reduces Your Humanity, Panders to Big Business… and Could Deprive You of Your Chance to Get Well (Page 280)

Part Six: Facing the New Frontier—What to Do Right Now!

Chapter 34: Spectators, Commentators, and Players—Why Some People Take Action and Get Well, While Others Stand On the Sidelines and Suffer (Page 286)

Chapter 35: Your New Beginning: What to Do Right Now! (Page 290)

Chapter 36: Frequently Asked Questions (Page 303)

Foreword

The natural and holistic methods described in this book have proven effective in helping patients with Lyme disease, and are equally effective in addressing other medical problems. Having personally overcome Lyme disease using such methods, I know firsthand. The techniques aim at identifying the various energetic disturbances in the human body, and supporting the innate defensive mechanisms to correct such disturbances. As a conventionally-trained medical doctor with over 30 years of experience in anesthesiology and pain management, as well as acupuncture and homeopathy, I am aware of the effectiveness and the limitations of both Western traditional medicine and complementary medicine. I have been blessed with the ability to use the best of both worlds.

We should not deny that many recent advances in Western medicine have been nothing short of amazing. Fascinating diagnostic procedures are now at hand, and new operative techniques such as laparoscopy and robotic surgery have added unprecedented safety to the surgical techniques. New medications are continuously introduced in an effort to improve their functionality. In emergencies and in life saving situations, Western medicine can offer miraculous approaches. However, the failure to identify the causes of the absolute majority of diseases has forced traditional Western medicine to become dependent on drug therapy that is only aiming at relief of symptoms.

There is no denial that diseases develop simply because the immune system has gone rogue. Unfortunately, the antibiotics, steroids, and immune-suppressants frequently used to treat both simple and complicated sicknesses further suppress the immune system. The tendency of the current medical treatments in Western medicine is to address the symptoms of the disease rather than addressing the cause. The failure of medical research to identify the cause of various sicknesses has prompted the medical community to seek avenues that offer comfort and restore some function.

Let us take an example of a person suffering from arthritis. As Western medicine is at a loss as to the actual cause, attention is directed at merely calming the symptoms. Pain alleviating medications and anti-inflammatory drugs can offer the patient some pain relief and temporarily improve the mobility of the joint, but at what expense? It is clear that this approach fails to influence the course of the disease. The disease process will continue unchecked and damage of the joint is inevitable. Total joint replacement is certainly on the horizon. Other current medical approaches include some drastic measures aimed at suppressing the immune system. Though this will considerably decrease the suffering of the individual, it can lead to serious and disastrous complications. Fortunately, we can seek simple measures to support regulation of the immune system that is naturally endowed with protecting our health. This book introduces the reader to some of the most fascinating approaches aiming at stabilizing our health and improving the functionality of our immune system *without* collateral damage.

Dr. Liebell began his training with me in 2009. He has taken the skills and knowledge I have shared with him in the field of homeopathic medicine and acupuncture, and combined it with his 25 years of existing expertise and experience in holistic health care to create a masterpiece. He is a crusader for the millions of sufferers of tick-borne illness, with a tireless commitment to helping as many people as humanly possible. This book elegantly explores the concepts of health and disease and offers suggestions of how we can proceed to address the effects of tick-borne infection, which is among the most difficult medical problems we face today.

Nader Soliman, M.D.
Integrative Medicine Center
Rockville, MD, USA
President, American Academy
of Medical Acupuncture (2003-2005)

Introduction

Congratulations on taking the first step towards recovering from the ravages of tick-triggered illness. This book debunks the many myths about Lyme disease, its diagnosis, and its treatment. To your delight, you will quickly realize this is <u>not</u> an academic medical book full of technical medical jargon. You will explore health and healing from a completely different perspective. Most importantly, when finished you will possess the knowledge of realistic hope for you to get better. It includes inspiring facts so powerful—*they astonished the doctors who discovered them!*

It is without excessive fanfare, exaggeration or drama that **Biting Back** tackles head on, one of the most critical, yet misunderstood and medically mismanaged epidemics of our time—in a manner contrary to existing approaches from both conventional *and* alternative medicine. The effects of all kinds of infections (not just Lyme *Borrelia*) result in a dazzling diversity of medical conditions for which doctors diagnose. It is not so much a matter of *mis*-diagnosis, but rather indifference or ignorance to the known root causes of such conditions.

This is not an academic medical textbook. Occasionally, I will use the term, Lyme disease, or simply "Lyme." Consider it a "buzz word," not a *scientific* term. You will notice I avoid the popular terminology associated with Lyme disease as much as possible. My terminology is tick-triggered illness. This is both accurate and important because many people never have "official" medical proof of Lyme *Borrelia* infection. I work outside the world of conventional health care, and even so-called *alternative* medicine. I take care of mostly long-suffering people, who are desperate for help... people who have been exploited and mistreated medically... people who do not have money to waste—because they've wasted way too much already—with atrocious results.

This book was not written for the lucky people who have responded *well* to conventional pharmaceutical medical care. My natural and holistic health care practice of 25 years (as of 2018) has not existed to serve those for whom antibiotics, herbs, and nutritional supplements have been successful. It is meant for everybody else! I cheer for any and all patients (and their doctors) who have succeeded through other approaches.

Do We Really Need *Another* Book on Lyme Disease?

There is no shortage of attention to the **topic** of Lyme disease. However, most books, films, articles, and news segments paint an unnecessarily frightening, bleak, and confusing picture. Their focus is on the history, politics, and controversy of the diagnosis of Lyme disease, and the ongoing debate over aggressive, risky, and costly long-term antibiotic therapy. It is riddled with conspiracy theory hype. None of that will drive you towards restoring your health. Do you need *another* Lyme disease history lesson, or chronicle of the public outrage over questionable blood tests and other medical mysteries? Talk about "beating a dead horse," how about another empathetic "misery-loves-company" memoir of mistreatment, and misdiagnosis? Are you seeking education in microbiology and the life cycle of ticks and bacteria?

With no disrespect meant to the well-intending authors, I submit that none of that will unshackle you from a life sentence of suffering. Sick and suffering people are lusting for effective treatment rather than having to learn how to doctor themselves. That is precisely why this is not a self-help book, but rather a **get help** book. You will be relieved that the burden of treatment is not on *you*.

2

If you were anticipating an assortment of tips to *cope* with Lyme disease, you will be sadly disappointed. You will not be enduring another misery-loves-company tale of woe. I will not be your tour guide through a trail of tears, nor will I subject you to yet another litany of antibiotic regimens, special diets, parasite cleanses, glutathione supplements, herbal medicines, removing dental fillings, "new age" philosophy, or eliminating every electronic device from your home. These are among the things various websites, support groups, books, herbalists, nutritionists, and doctors have perhaps convinced you that you must do.

This book was designed primarily for sufferers of tick-triggered illness for whom aggressive long-term antibiotic treatment and other Lyme protocols have failed. However, it is also for those who wish to avoid the obscene costs and risks of such treatments, and pursue easy, safe, and affordable holistic natural treatment right from start. It is a no-nonsense and no-holds-barred guide for both existing patients and prospective patients. It is also for progressive-thinking doctors, who are interested in learning how to help sick and suffering people in a manner beyond their wildest dreams and expectations.

Today we have doctors who have designated themselves specialists in Lyme disease. The public calls them *"Lyme Literate medical doctors"* (LLMD). Despite more of the scientific community declaring the impending doom of the antibiotics era, these physicians aggressively prescribe long-term antibiotic treatment. This includes cases where no medical evidence of active bacterial infection exists. Considering the ominous specter of globally-expanding antibiotic-resistant infection, and the risks of serious side effects and complications (including death) from antibiotic usage, there has never been a more critical time for implementing radically different strategies.

All Doctors Should Be Lyme Disease Savvy

I applaud all practitioners who help sufferers of Lyme disease. However, I cringe at the LLMD terminology. There is no such medical degree. If anything, reference should be made to Lyme *ignorant* doctors. With this in mind, if you are seeking advice on how to find a doctor, who is willing to prescribe you indefinite courses of antibiotics—you would best return this book, or give it to somebody else. Give it to somebody who is ready to do something revolutionary—something *beyond* out-of-the-box.

Victims of tick-triggered illness are brainwashed to believe a variety of regimens, rituals, and treatments are absolutely necessary. They just cannot let go. For many, the first (and often most difficult) step on the road to wellness is to *unlearn* many of these things they have accepted as Lyme disease gospel. The public has been convinced that the human immune system is not capable of beating *Borrelia* bacteria without long-term antibiotics and other risky, expensive, controversial, and complicated treatments. Others are convinced that nobody can really get better at all—Lyme can only be *managed*. The public is further confused by doctors, who create controversy by declaring that there is no such thing as *chronic* Lyme disease. Perhaps it is easier to insist that an illness doesn't exist than to effectively deal with it. Despite its many magnificent achievements, conventional medicine has failed abysmally to fulfill its promise with regards to Lyme disease.

Biting Back proposes a radically different health care approach— designed precisely for those who have become collateral damage from a medical system that inhumanely permits you to suffer the inhumanity of spiraling down the abyss of dozens of different diagnoses and drugs, only to be sicker than when you started. You will learn exactly what needs to be done (and why), and of equal (or perhaps greater) importance, what *not* to do. If you decide to pursue what is recommended in this book, you stand an excellent chance of joining an elite group of people who share the most impressive and extraordinary recovery success stories in the country… all without a single drug, herb, or complex dietary regimen.

Knowledge Is Truly Power— Only If One Takes Action!

People hunger desperately for truth. Hype and hysteria have reached epidemic proportions. Style massively exceeds substance. In this book, you will acquire authentic information to drive yourself towards recovery from chronic tick-triggered illness. You will be gently guided without exaggeration, or unrealistic promises of single-solution "miracle cures." Stunning as it might seem, much of what you are about to learn is *not* new. Its components have been published in medical journals and other science publications! Yet this knowledge seems to be scarcely applied in practice, or available to the general public.

My responsibility is to help people to get healthier. I call my holistic treatment approach the *Bio-energetic Individual Treatment Equation*©. It is something so different that few doctors are currently willing to do it. I have written this book, in part to encourage more doctors to "get aboard the train"—for the sake of the public! I am determined to become an unstoppable fighting force for victims of tick-triggered illness across the country, and confront the mysteries, while avoiding the wedge issues of antibiotics, politics, blood tests, and high-risk medical practices.

Why am I doing this?

This is a very personal and passionate mission (you'll learn why in Chapter One). When one discovers something important enough, the goal is to make sure everyone who needs it can get it—not just the rich, entitled, or health-insured. The tremendous joy felt cannot be quantified when it comes to helping restore quality of life to people for whom all previous attempts by other doctors, treatment protocols, and facilities have failed. This book has been lovingly crafted to serve the suffering souls who have been cast aside by other doctors as hopeless, or drugged into oblivion.

There is undeniable pleasure in silencing skeptics. However, it is not due to *ego*, but rather because there is no greater reward than witnessing the progressive, real, and lasting improvements my patients naturally achieve. I treasure the rare privilege to consistently witness firsthand the extraordinary healing capacity of the human body. You will see, sprinkled throughout this book, many testimonial letters from my patients. I appreciate their willingness to put their experiences in print—to help others have the same opportunity for a better life that they now relish. Testimonials serve as encouragement that there is realistic hope for you too. My patients' stories of triumph will inspire you for the chance of duplicating their success. These letters are all true and accurate, and were provided willingly, without any compensation offered in return.

Unlike those you see in late night infomercials, they actually *do* represent typical results. It is unfortunate that many folks are too shy to write, or appear on camera, thus some of the best success stories go unpublished. I respect that many others wish to remain anonymous because public knowledge of their illness could affect their employment or personal relationships. Some people prefer simply to keep their medical problems private. With this in mind, some of the testimonials include first name and last initial only. The truth about these testimonials is that it is really not *me* they are praising, but rather the magnificent techniques, technologies, and knowledge I have accumulated, along with my tireless dedication for producing extraordinary and consistent results during the past twenty-three years.

I do not profess that these testimonials constitute academic research or medical proof. They serve as referrals, recommendations, or user reviews in the manner that one might explore such for purchasing various goods or services. I cannot state more boldly and strongly that I do not claim a "cure" for chronic Lyme disease, as other authors and doctors may do. My experience and expertise is in holistic, natural, and supportive treatment, which enables people to recover through their own built-in natural healing mechanisms. Holistic doctors suffer the often insurmountable task of delivering concrete proof of results. Although case studies may be academically published, individual results cannot be easily quantified. Nevertheless, referrals pour in. My patients have been perfectly happy to go by the rave reviews of others, rather than the dogma of self-appointed "authorities," who have done nothing but let them down.

The Ranting Of a Lyme Disease Rebel

You have been duped. Our health care system has systematically brainwashed you to believe pain and illness are *normal* and inevitable parts of life. They doom you to "pain management" to deal with physical and mental illness that is largely blamed on genetics, age, and bad luck. Your future health picture is painted with an abundance of visits to doctors, hospitals, and pharmacies. Your other option is to just accept it and learn to live with pain and illness. The conventional wisdom is that there is no hope beyond prescribing you drugs to keep you more comfortable. Health is not a common commodity in America. Nor is living life where problems can be naturally prevented, or handled with drug-free methods.

The amount of chronic pain suffered in America is staggering. Conventional medical approaches rarely, if ever make people *healthier*, nor do they always achieve their desired result. Medicines are prescribed to treat diagnoses rather than *people*. Doctors eagerly dispatch their bountiful supply of "designer drugs for designer conditions." Such prescriptions are gleefully provided to those who *qualify* with the right symptoms. In my opinion, this practice is based on guidelines intended to be the *minimal* level of care a doctor can provide. In all fairness, bringing relief to chronic pain sufferers is an arduous task for doctors—even when armed with heavy duty medications. Consider how significant an accomplishment it is to bring blessed relief to people *without* drugs! That is my thrill and passion. Pain banishment beats pain *management*, hands down!

"It must be true... I saw it on the Internet!"

Victims of tick-triggered illness tend to be thorough in their investigation. Why? Because they are *forced* to! Perhaps in a more competent and caring medical system, the *patient* should not have to be the one to research and ask for diagnostic tests, or suggest a possible diagnosis. The *Internet* should not have to be the means to arrive at a tentative diagnosis of Lyme disease. Doctors and medical researchers should be well aware that microorganisms are agents of disease, and consider such causes.

Past generations widely believed if they saw it on television, or read it in the newspaper—it must be true. Of course, this was never accurate thinking. It is infinitely worse today thanks to the Internet. Today, anybody can broadcast opinions and views on the Internet. Honesty and accuracy are not required for anybody

8

to pose as a journalist or expert. What this means is that intelligent people and not-so-intelligent get equal media "airtime." The less intelligent appear to be *more* aggressive and louder-voiced than those with legitimate experience, skills, wisdom, and judgment. As a result, the loudmouths, know-it-alls, and opinionated ignoramuses get the lion's share of attention.

Case in point is the attitude of doctors who scold their patients if they have the audacity to bring up Lyme disease. Are those doctors compassionate, wise, and experienced? No. They are the ones who do not read books or medical journals, and tell people they have fibromyalgia or whatever condition they like to give as a one-size-fits-all diagnosis...with a prescription of a designer drug to match. They accept that a positive Western Blot, or a doctor eye-witnessed "bull's eye" rash serve as the only criteria for diagnosing Lyme disease (if they are even aware of that). These are the prototypical Lyme-*ignorant* doctors. Ignorance is abundant and doesn't cost a penny! Set on the world's stage of the Internet, misinformation is more plentiful and accessible than ever in history.

We have heard the mantra, "You can't fix stupid." There's a lot of stupid on the Web. Experience, expertise, effectiveness, and wisdom seem to be the exception—not the rule. These sought-after attributes come with a price. They are the result of commitment, effort, experimentation, investigation, discernment, and financial investment. As a consumer, you are faced with the task of choosing between intelligence and ignorance every day. The real task is in figuring out who is who! Get-rich-quick schemes, alleged overnight cures and "miracle drugs" are thrust before you—enticing you and mesmerizing you. Their raw power can overwhelm you, interfering with your ability to developing the insight and good judgment to take a careful look at what is currently going on, what has gone on in the past (and the results of such), which enables wiser decisions.

9

"My Way... or the Highway"?

The primary tools of conventional Western medicine are drugs, surgery, and physical therapy. Anything else is denigrated as "alternative medicine." This is equally unfortunate as it is preposterous. In mathematics, there are usually numerous ways to arrive at a solution to a problem. The same applies to health care, where various treatments, techniques, systems, philosophies, sciences, and arts can enable recovery from illness and injury. Nevertheless, challenging American mainstream medicine's "crown jewel," antibiotics on *any* level constitutes medical blasphemy. Certainly, antibiotics are one of the greatest developments in the history of medicine. There is no disputing they have saved countless lives and brought blessed relief to countless millions. Unfortunately, due to many decades of misuse and abuse, the nuclear bomb that was designed to annihilate enemy bacteria has backfired. Despite a rising mountain of scientific evidence that killing the beneficial bacteria along with the harmful has dire consequences—the prescriptions persist prolifically. This is especially pertinent in consideration of long-term antibiotic usage, a practice for which science has not validated (to my knowledge) as safe and warranted.

Medical professionals maintain a love-hate relationship with antibiotics. Some view them as lifesaving pharmaceutical miracles, while others condemn them as representing all that is wrong with modern medicine. The fact is that any substance that is capable of altering human biochemical pathways will also bring unintended consequences. Sufferers of tick-triggered illness commonly wonder to what degree their symptoms are the result of infection versus the side effects of antibiotics.

The bottom line is one cannot promote life by killing. Antibiotics are designed for bacterial genocide. If only our enemy was the entire bacterial kingdom. It is not. Most bacterial species residing in our bodies are helpful and necessary, if not harmless. More collateral damage results from overuse and inappropriate use of the drugs than ever anticipated, dating back to the dawn of the antibiotic era. The realization of antibiotic-resistant bacteria is not new, nor is it challenged scientifically. Global epidemics such as methicillin-resistant *Staphylococcus aureus* (MRSA) merely scratch the surface of the problem.

Nevertheless, mainstream medicine conversely clings to a militaristic view—a war against bacteria, demonstrated by its single-minded philosophy of antibiotic treatment for Lyme *Borrelia*, and any other microbes that stand in its way. Even if the smokescreen of controversy over the diagnosis and acceptance of *chronic* Lyme disease could clear away—antibiotic treatment would still be the focus of treatment. Considering that many top scientists have been saying that the era of antibiotics has *ended*, it could not be more timely and critical to look to other approaches.

Mainstream Medicine Has Had Their Chance to Handle Chronic Lyme Disease... but Have Blown it!

Our health care system is broken. I am not talking about insurance, but rather the actual *care* itself. If we dig deep enough, and gaze far beyond what is conventional, contemporary, or traditional there is a massive amount of overlooked, underused, and forgotten health wisdom to be found. There have been numerous legitimate and progressive health breakthroughs that have been systematically and unscrupulously ignored by the gatekeepers of mainstream medicine (usually for lack of profitability). I have pursued such wisdom throughout my career. Finally, after years of frustration, desperately seeking solutions for chronic tick-triggered illness, I stumbled upon the very breakthrough that those afflicted with it desperately need. I too, at first thought it was too good to be true. It seemed too easy, too simple, and too inexpensive.

11

Serving those who have been ravaged by the effects of tick-triggered illness has become my passion and my life's work. I am not being overly dramatic, or cliché, in saying that you are going to learn about life-changing health secrets that will blow your mind. What is even more exciting is that because it is a natural and holistic *wellness*-based system, there is not a shred of Lyme disease controversy, nor is there a political or financial agenda over which to lose sleep. This is a huge development! Plus, it is not a bank account-siphoning ordeal like many patients suffer through various so-called Lyme specialty clinics.

Tragedy Trumps Triumph?

We are peppered with television talk shows, news segments, and documentaries on Lyme disease that showcase the same tired arguments over antibiotics and blood tests. The patients are struggling and suffering. The doctors are portrayed as tragic heroes—persecuted for their selfless crusade to bring antibiotics indefinitely, to those in need. This hardly seems logical as the world teeters ominously on the edge of the end of the antibiotics era.

Must history always repeat itself? Are we not supposed to learn from mistakes? The public has little exposure to legitimate stories of *triumph*! You will be shocked and delighted when you grasp the reality that the burden of chronic tick-triggered illness can likely be lifted from you. The torment and heartbreak that it has caused you, which has been the bane of your existence, can realistically come to an end. It is information for you to devour—a shock to the status quo. Consistently witnessing the magnificent healing power of the human body is an ongoing awe-inspiring experience. The secret is so amazingly simple to have done that it requires almost no effort on your part. Yet it is so powerful, it could enable your body to naturally overcome chronic pain and illness after all else has failed.

Intrigued? You should be—most victims of tick-triggered illness who have correctly implemented the *Bio-energetic Individual Treatment Equation©* have succeeded… **Now it's your turn!** My intention is to provide you with an experience that you will look back on as a turning point in your life. When your natural healing capacity demonstrates its raw power like never before, you see a "new universe" of health care with a new, inner vision. When your ability to overcome chronic illness takes a quantum leap, you will know in your heart that your future is secure. The treatment is so simple, easy, effective, and so inexpensive that it has no *corporate financial value*. There is no drug to patent, or stock to sell on the open market. This is purely a "grassroots" effort. The results people achieve are real. What do I mean by "real?" True health and healing is when your body progressively makes improvements from the inside out—through its own inborn healing power, rather than drugs (and/or herbs) masking symptoms.

Scientific discovery has always teetered between ignorance and knowledge. What we humans think is one hundred percent certainly true today can be disproven in a heartbeat tomorrow. Before microscopes enabled us to see the hidden world of living things, we concocted all kinds of mystical explanations for diseases. The *Borrelia* bacterium as a cause of the symptoms of Lyme disease was at one time unknown too. The farther we move away from nature—the more we must rely on human intellect. This can be either good or bad. Mainstream medicine has scared us away from various healthful practices that are essential to human health.

Too Good to be True?

I accept the reality that the majority of people will "blow this off" because it sounds too good to be true. Most will ignore it, and continue to suffer, consuming a fortune in symptom-masking, side-effect-causing drugs, and/or "Herxing" on herbs and Rife machines for the rest of their lives. By writing about this topic, and promoting a unique holistic *wellness* system, I am going out on a limb. I'm risking public and professional ridicule. If this approach *fails* to deliver results, the reputation that I've built over 23 years would go by the wayside. Do you think I would risk tarnishing my reputation with something that was anything but effective? No way! So settle back and read on. You are in for a heck of a ride!

Part One:

Crushing the Controversies and Conundrums

"Healing is a matter of time, but it is sometimes also a matter of opportunity." - Hippocrates

Chapter 1

How a Frazzled Mother-of-Three, Desperate for Answers and Losing Hope... *Conquered* Chronic Lyme Disease... <u>Without</u> Antibiotics, Herbs, or Complicated Diets

A growing number of people around the country are raving about their own recoveries, thanks to a very special person, named Sheila. For several years, Sheila suffered severe fatigue, mood swings, joint and muscle pain, heart palpitations, memory problems, and many other symptoms. Every day was a struggle to take care of her three very young children and manage her home. Sheila was hardly a 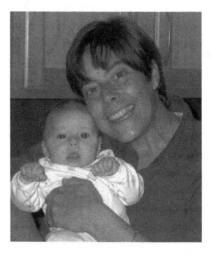 couch potato. She played high school varsity softball, basketball, and volleyball, as well as college tennis. But sports became completely out of the question due to her mysterious illness.

Sheila never had the supposedly classic bull's eye rash associated with Lyme disease, nor did she recall seeing a tick. No doctor ever suggested a Lyme blood test. But one day, Sheila asked for it herself ... by *accident*! She had read a lot about West Nile virus and thought perhaps it could be at the root of her problems. At her check-up, Sheila was actually thinking, and intending to ask the doctor to test for West Nile virus, but the words got scrambled up in her brain (as they often did), and they came out of her mouth as *"Lyme disease!"*

What a strange stroke of luck it was. Thankfully, Sheila's general physician was open-minded and not too egotistical to accept a suggestion from his patient. He ordered a blood test, and shockingly, it was indeed positive for Lyme disease! Sheila was both shocked and thrilled at the same time. At least she had some sort of explanation for some of her symptoms. Still, it was only the beginning of a long and painful odyssey—but ultimately with a happy ending, which I will be sharing with you. You see, the mission of this book is to empower <u>you</u> to experience the same happy ending as Sheila!

Once Sheila was officially diagnosed with Lyme disease, she was prescribed a long course of antibiotics, with the expectations that she would return to her original fit and healthy self. Wishful thinking as it was, the antibiotic treatment was an abysmal failure. The drugs tore up Sheila's stomach, and many of her symptoms got progressively *worse*—even though it allegedly "cured" her Lyme disease. Over a period of several years, Sheila tried all kinds of "alternative" medicine treatments, like the highly-touted vitamin C and salt protocol. She tried frequency generator treatments, as well as herbal medicines, colonics, nutritional cleanses, and other treatments. But they were equally ineffective, leaving her discouraged, miserable, frustrated, and desperate for relief. The only thing that kept Sheila in one piece was frequent chiropractic treatment (mostly for her upper neck). But finally, after much perseverance…

Sheila DEFEATED Lyme Disease!

She received the treatment that she now knows in her heart, victims of chronic tick-triggered illness *really* need. It was a defining moment in Sheila's life! She realized it was her mission in life—her responsibility to help others with the same affliction. With her health and vitality restored, Sheila was able to work again. She took a position at a holistic health clinic where she could serve as a role model and coach—to help others get their lives back, just like she did.

Perhaps this sounds like a story right out of Hollywood. You know, the tragedy stricken, near death victim who finds a miracle cure close to her final hour. The difference is that this is a <u>true</u> story. You see, Sheila is my *wife*! And the holistic health clinic is my office. If you take Sheila's story to heart, you could possibly be rewarded beyond your wildest dreams. In the beginning, Sheila's situation seemed hopeless. In addition to other practitioners, I tried everything I knew how to do. But all I could do was manage some of her symptoms (I am her chiropractor!).

Was she going to have to learn to live with her problems? Was Sheila going *crazy?* It was terrifying. I learned that many a poor soul has been sent to the psychiatrist—their physicians never considered or believed that Lyme disease could easily have been at the heart of their "mental problems." I read a study published in 2002 in the *American Journal of Psychiatry*. It revealed that 33% of the psychiatric patients had signs of Lyme infection! Top psychiatrists have acknowledged that Lyme disease can possibly contribute to the development of any psychiatric disorder. One might think this would be common knowledge, and that every psychiatrist would consider it. But it does not seem to be the case at all.

Sheila has been an inspiration to many. Lyme disease victims from around the country have called to speak with her for her guidance and empathy, but most important to share the secrets of her success... which is now *their* success too! The fact is there really *are* all kinds of overlooked health secrets. I'm not being cliché here. There is a massive amount of underused and forgotten wisdom about health and health care. I have proudly spent the last 25 years pursuing such knowledge and skills, and using it to help people who were told they *couldn't* get well.

Taking Sheila's situation into my own hands was necessary. I could not passively rely on the advice of overwhelmed and uninformed doctors to save my wife. Nobody was as concerned with her welfare as I was. Most doctors are restricted to brief visits with their patients. The reality in the *business* of modern medicine is that most doctors either cannot or will not devote much time and thought to your situation. I learned to be very leery of "conventional wisdom" in health care. Why? Because our long-broken mainstream medical system has not produced results to be proud of, or to trust when it comes to chronic illness in general, and certainly not tick-triggered illness. My experience was to get current on whatever the conventional wisdom was on Lyme, and run for the hills! I sought out advice that ran *contrary* to what everyone else was saying! I was resolved to be smart about it, and not believe everything I read, and not latch onto the first "miracle cure" I came across. I wanted the full story—the untold story. I knew it was out there.

Primum Non Nocere: "First, Do No Harm." - Unknown

Chapter 2

If You are Losing the Battle, Switch the Battlefield!

By practicing holistic wellness methods that are not dependent upon direct diagnosis or treatment of Lyme disease, I stand clear of the controversy—while providing outstanding outcomes. I am neutral (like Switzerland) when it comes to Lyme wars. Other doctors, politicians, insurance companies, medical boards, and pharmaceutical companies can fight their hostile uphill battles. Their polarized disagreements are preventing people from a chance at health and happiness. I pity those who choose to continue suffering—exclusively putting their faith in conventional medicine (a system that has failed them miserably), waiting for them to give the "thumbs up" to another approach. It would be delightful if everybody could simply take antibiotics to recover from the ravages of chronic tick-triggered illness. If this were the case, *Biting Back* would never have been even conceived.

It is not a matter of the *Bio-energetic Individual Treatment Equation* being natural—but rather that it is effective. The secrets to my patients' success has nothing whatsoever to do with the philosophy or methods of *any* of the organizations currently associated with the controversy and politics of Lyme disease including: *Centers for Disease Control* (CDC), *Infectious Disease Society of America* (IDSA), *International Lyme and Associated Diseases Society* (ILADS), *American Medical Association,* and the *U.S. Food and Drug Administration* (FDA). State medical boards, university and private research facilities, pharmaceutical companies, various Lyme disease groups, and individual practitioners are also part of the ugly mix.

20

My proclamation to you is that you are NOT obligated to participate. I am not fighting *their* fight. You do not have to either!

What good has it done you? The clock is ticking. It is *your* life that needs repairing. The American health care system is not *your* battlefield. You are not obligated to fight "Lyme wars." It is not *your* job to improve doctors' understanding or acceptance of chronic Lyme disease, nor is *your* responsibility to develop research studies. It should not be *your* job to convince the doctor why you are sick, and how to treat your illness.

There once was a time that I naively assumed rheumatologists, neurologists, infectious disease specialists, immunologists, and general physicians had Lyme disease covered. How wrong I was. Helping chronic pain sufferers has always been my expertise—but chronic Lyme disease… seriously? I am a doctor of chiropractic, and I am also licensed in acupuncture. I could never have predicted that one day it would be *my* mission—my responsibility to help victims of tick-triggered illness.

Core BITE Principle: I refer to my patients as <u>victims of tick-triggered Illness</u>. For many, there is no laboratory diagnostic medical proof of active *Borrelia burgdorferi* (or other infection). This is of no consequence, since I do not treat infectious disease, nor do I portray myself as a "Lyme literate" medical doctor (LLMD).

I utilize a comprehensive holistic approach that is liberating people from a life of chronic pain, fatigue and dozens of other symptoms—without any medication. It is NOT a direct treatment for Lyme disease, or any other medical condition. At first, this may be a difficult concept to grasp. It is my duty to guide you out of the darkness… to "see the light" of better health.

21

It is critical to understand that the task-at-hand is to "turbo-charge" your body—so *it* can beat tick-triggered illness. **My proposal to you is to start from scratch**. Put behind you whatever your beliefs have been about what you have been told you need to do. Come to terms with the fact that whatever methods that have failed you in your quest for health must be buried in the past, at least for now. None of it will likely support you moving forward. I feel it is safe to assume that since you are reading this book that you have attempted other evaluation and treatment methods without satisfactory results.

However, if you change your approach, you could give yourself a new lease on life. This is a priceless concept that's critical to grasp--especially when what you have been trying to do to restore your health has been *failing*. My mission is to give you a new lease on life, and to do so, I must effectively help you un-learn many concepts that perhaps you have been clinging on to—despite their lack of effectiveness. These are the battlefields on which you have been losing the war against chronic illness and pain. Let's explore them together!

The Diagnosis Battlefield

Those who have recovered from chronic tick-triggered illness by applying the *Bio-energetic Individual Treatment Equation©* understand that conventional medical diagnosis was not what led them down the path to wellness. Diagnosis of Lyme disease in the conventional medical sense had little-to-nothing to do with restoring their health. Much experience has taught me that an emotional attachment to the diagnosis of Lyme disease has held people back from getting the care they really needed. Has the assignment of a *name* for your condition been your salvation? Unless you have been one of the lucky people who got immediately diagnosed with Lyme, took antibiotics, and never had a problem—I suspect it is highly unlikely. It is pitiful for me to consistently hear new patients tell me their tragic tale of traveling from doctor-to-doctor to find one who was willing to officially diagnose Lyme disease. Blood test interpretation and controversy—we do not fight on the diagnosis "battlefield" with the *Bio-energetic Individual Treatment Equation*! It does not enter into "the equation." You will understand much more about this by reading the chapter on diagnosis.

The Lyme Disease <u>Treatment</u> Battlefield

Nearly all patients who have come to the Liebell Clinic have been administered numerous Lyme disease treatments from various physicians. This includes antibiotics, herbs, nutritional, and many other Lyme protocols. The battle against Lyme disease has been the agenda of both patients and doctors. Bacterial warfare has been their battlefield of choice.

I provide the opportunity for patients and prospective patients who have failed to get well (and stay well) to switch the battlefield, pronto! A single bacterial species, Lyme *Borrelia* is *not* the true enemy. **Dysfunction of one's immune system to fight not just *Borrelia*, but countless other harmful microbes (that cannot be killed by antibiotic "bombs") is the ultimate problem!** I repeatedly state that I do not fight Lyme wars because I never enter the battlefield in the first place. Call me Switzerland! Supporting natural regulation of the body's defenses is the name of the game. This fundamental *Bio-Energetic Individual Treatment Equation* (BITE) principle is detailed in many chapters.

The Nutrition Battlefield

Nobody likes to admit making poor choices. But it seems people tend to cling to them particularly when large amounts of money have been spent. Patients commonly enter my office hoisting a sack of vitamins and mineral supplements, herbs, enzymes, antioxidants, and other pills. They are uncertain of what to do with them; they've paid for them, but they have not

23

been helping much at all. Often is the case that the patient has been taking their supplements for *years*—and do not feel comfortable without them, despite having felt no benefit from their consumption. This is another example of fighting on the wrong battlefield. Perhaps you, like many of my patients, have spent thousands of dollars on nutritional supplements. I am certain that a big part of the problem is that people have become too comfortable with nutritional supplementation. The perception that poor nutrition is the chief cause of most illnesses is in my opinion, something that leads people down the wrong path.

I have always been an ardent advocate of nutrition, exercise, and other health practices. I encourage good nutrition (covered in a later chapter) as part of the wellness equation, but it is not the critical recovery factor for most patients. So many patients I have encountered lived incredibly healthy lifestyles—both nutritionally and with regards to exercise and other practices. But tick-borne illness and its numerous consequences still did them in! It was not a lack of nutrition.

The Detox and Cleanse Battlefield

Many a victim of Lyme has waged the war against toxins. Perhaps some small battles have been won. However, the forceful cleansing of toxins appears to consistently come up short. This is hardly to say that keeping one's body as clean and clear as possible is not a fine idea. In the chapter on detoxification, you will understand why trying to aggressively purge toxins can be a poor choice. We are all constantly fighting a battle against toxic chemicals. It is true that we are bombarded with more poisons than any time in human history. However, this does not mean it is a wise move to try to vigorously expel them from our bodies. Will this improve one's ability to develop strength against Lyme bacteria, viruses, or other pathogens?

Perhaps, but it is a "battlefield" that so many chronic Lyme sufferers have returned from battered, bruised, and brutalized in bitter defeat.

With the *Bio-energetic Individual Treatment Equation*© we seek to support the body to regulate its own normal and healthy detoxification systems of the body that functioned adequately prior to tick-borne infection. We put our trust in the time-tested human immune system that with a bit of support, is "armed and ready to do battle," as it has for as long as humans have walked the planet. It is not a matter of faith. For those enlightened doctors, who have had the privilege to consistently witness the true healing capabilities of the human body, it is simply a matter of expectation based on experience.

Part Two:

Debunking Diagnosis Disasters

Iceman Murder Mystery

Just in case you think Lyme disease is a recent phenomenon, guess again. On September 26, 2011, PBS aired their exciting NOVA special, *Iceman Murder Mystery.* It featured the forensic investigation of a mummified corpse pulled from a glacier in the Italian Alps. Through autopsy, scientists discovered that "Ötzi the Iceman" who died over 5,000 years ago had Lyme disease!

"Those who merely study and treat the effects of disease are like those who imagine that they can drive away the winter by brushing the snow off the door… It is not the snow that causes winter, but the winter that causes the snow." - Paracelsus (1493-1542)

Chapter 3

Borrelia Band Blunders & the Dangerous Delusion of Diagnosis

According to the *National Institutes of Health* (NIH), there's actually only one way to be 100% certain of a correct diagnosis—the only sign or symptom unique to Lyme disease: the "bull's eye" rash that sometimes follows an infectious tick bite. It can show up between 3 and 30 days afterwards. The rash usually lasts between 3 and 5 weeks. It is certainly possible that immediate antibiotic treatment upon noticing it might prevent a lifetime of needless suffering. Blood tests are unnecessary if you develop such a rash following a tick bite. Doctors are supposed to diagnose Lyme based on a combination of detailed medical history (including past knowledge of tick bites) and physical exam. According to the CDC, laboratory tests can be *helpful* but are not recommended when a patient has an expanding red rash following a tick bite.

Lyme Diagnosis: No Rash = No Proof

What if you have never seen a tick on your body? What if you do not have an allergic sensitivity to tick bites? Clearly, many people do not develop *any* sort of expanding red rash (erythema migrans)—let alone the supposedly classic bull's eye rash. The same is true with mosquito bites. Not everybody suffers an itchy allergic response. A person could be infected by a mosquito bite without having any telltale sign of being bitten. There are beekeepers who are immune to the stings of their

27

honey-making friends, while others can go into anaphylactic shock from the same! The opposite can be true. One can be allergic to a bug's bite, but have strong immunity against infectious microbes transmitted by it. The bottom line is that the bull's eye is bull!

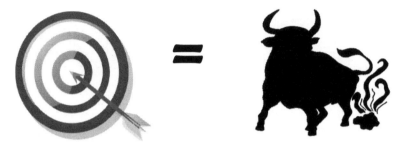

I see little reason to call it a classic sign of Lyme disease when so few Lyme victims I have encountered had developed one. My wife, Sheila never had one, and neither did I (yes, I have had Lyme disease, too).

Beware the Blood Tests

The *Centers for Disease Control* (CDC) currently state 300,000 new cases of Lyme disease arise each year—tenfold of their previous reporting. My suspicion is the actual figure is many times that amount since the established blood tests miss perhaps half or more cases of infection. Many people have reported a downward spiral in their health following tick bites, even though blood tests results were normal. The diagnostic criteria for medically confirming Lyme disease by means of the Western Blot blood test are very firm. The CDC requires either 5 out of 10 possible *Borrelia* bands in one group, or 2 out of 3 in the other to confirm a positive test. These bands reflect an antibody immune response to either the presence or past presence of the bacterial infection. There are several well-known laboratories that perform the tests. Many patients who have failed to get a positive test will seek confirmation by paying considerably higher fees to a West Coast lab that tests for more strains of *Borrelia* than others. Either way, it is clear that blood tests are woefully unreliable to confirm the presence of *Borrelia* infection. They are equally woeful for measuring progress after antibiotic treatment!

Imagine how many people must be suffering the effects of tick-borne infection, but don't know it. As a result, it is neither tested for, nor reported statistically. The findings of *Virginia's Lyme Task Force* appointed by the Governor of Virginia stated that no blood test is capable of ruling out Lyme disease! Diagnosis of Lyme is a matter of a doctor's opinion when there has been neither a bull's eye rash, nor a positive blood test.

Why Lyme Obsession Drives You *Away* from the Your Road to Wellness

Recovery achieved through applying the *Bio-energetic Individual Treatment Equation*© is not the result of trying to definitively diagnose and kill *Borrelia*. Obsession with Lyme can hold you back from recovery. This single bacterial species is *not* your arch nemesis. Your immune system is indeed capable of beating it—with the right support! Tick-borne microbes did not just show up recently on planet Earth, nor have they been ruining the lives of every person exposed to them.

It is vital to ask yourself the question, "Will being formally diagnosed with Lyme disease enable me to get well?" What if I have already taken plenty of antibiotics?" Becoming qualified to be part of the statistics hardly casts off the shackles of chronic illness. Are we interested in proving that Lyme disease is an epidemic? Is it our mission to prove that *Borrelia* is the root of all evil? Or are we searching for the road to better health? I pity those who seek validation of their illness as their primary goal.

29

We applaud the doctors, who declare patients to be suffering from Lyme disease (and/or the publicized co-infections). However, there is a dark side to this revelation.

Core BITE Principle: You are NOT your symptoms. You are NOT a statistic, nor are you Lyme disease. The sooner you understand this, the sooner you can get well.

For many, it is not so much the actual Lyme infection, but rather the label itself that creates the stumbling block to better health. If you receive effective treatment, your body heals itself, your symptoms fade away, and you experience health and vitality once again—will you care what your condition was *named*? Will you care what anybody thinks? My advice is to free yourself from the distractions that come from the simplistic and inaccurate assumption that everything that ails you is the result of Lyme disease and the publicized co-infections. If you do not, you confine yourself to a potentially endless pursuit for the cure for it. Overcoming possible chronic infection from *Borrelia* is just one part of a much bigger equation. **Do not make Lyme disease your identity!**

When we utilize a whole-body, wellness-based approach to treatment, the name of your condition or syndrome does not matter. I do not treat infectious disease, nor do I treat the Lyme disease, MS, peripheral neuropathy, fibromyalgia, or any other diagnosis. I treat PEOPLE who suffer pain, fatigue, neurological symptoms, and other problems. A diagnosis may be a helpful shortcut, as we investigate for the means to get better. We want to use non-pharmaceutical approaches to support your body so your immune system functions better—so *it* eliminates microbial causes of whatever your condition is categorized as, and to support natural healing and halt further degeneration.

"To raise new questions, new possibilities, to regard old problems from a new angle, requires creative imagination and marks real advance in science." - Albert Einstein

Chapter 4

Why Conventional Western Medicine is a <u>Lemon</u> for Lyme

Conventional Western medicine has been dramatically successful in defeating many illnesses. There is no disputing that acute cases of Lyme disease may be resolved by prompt antibiotic treatment. That, however, is not the subject matter of this book. In fact, neither is the *diagnosis* of Lyme disease. I shall explain. With the conventional American medical approach, the goal is generally for the doctor to quickly make a diagnosis (name your condition) and provide whatever medical treatment has been established as appropriate or standard. Diagnosis is based upon signs, symptoms and some of the patient's background. The success rate is generally excellent when it comes to promptly and correctly treating *acute* conditions and emergency situations. The diagnosis is of utmost importance. It is a necessary process to "put out the fire." However, this approach is poorly suited for *chronic* pain and illness.

A major flaw in the American health care system is the attempt to use the same treatment methods for both acute and chronic health problems. Chronic illness is not comparable to a fire that needs to be extinguished. It must be viewed in a completely different manner in order to succeed. With chronic and complex illness, it is scandalously insufficient for a doctor to merely name the illness with a single diagnosis. Barely any attention is paid to the patient beyond the signs and symptoms.

The patient's entire health picture and circumstances do not get investigated thoroughly within the framework of their body. Each individual symptom or diagnosis is regarded as a separate problem for which a separate medication is prescribed. This is a major shortcoming of conventional Western medicine

There are usually MANY underlying causes of chronic pain, fatigue, neurological symptoms, psychiatric disorders, and other problems. All agents of disease, triggers, and other factors must be investigated and considered within the context of the whole human being. That's what holistic medicine is all about! The diagnosis remains useful, but becomes less important. You will soon understand that the secret to success for those who have applied the *Bio-energetic Individualized Treatment Equation* (BITE) was shifting their focus *away* from the diagnosis and treatment of Lyme disease!

Americans spend more per capita on health care than any other country, yet have little to show for their enormous investment. Ongoing treatment that serves to manage chronic pain and treat symptoms is crippling to our nation's economy. It does not account for the fact that chronic illness now far surpasses acute illness. Our health care system scarcely rewards people who take measures to ensure better health. In fact, we are punished. Most measures of health prevention are not compensated for by medical insurance. There is little financial reward for those spending extra money on higher-quality food, natural health maintenance treatments, gym memberships, and wellness-based programs. Imagine if all Americans received substantial tax deductions for *not* needing medical care? Legitimate preventative measures are rarely paid for by medical insurance. "Wellness" evaluations may have merit, but they are not proactive measures that actually strengthen one's health.

We do not really have a health care system at all. It is a disease and injury care system only. One of the deterrents to implementing change is that there is a fortune to be made in keeping people comfortable while they remain *sick*. This is pharmaceutical medicine's wheelhouse. The holistic and natural wellness model of health care unfortunately does not conform to the system. Addressing the whole person, and accounting for each person's health lifestyle, genetic makeup, and other influences takes effort and concentration. This does not fit the 15-minute doctor visit/insurance coverage model of care. The acute symptom treatment model of medicine fits like a glove!

Self-Diagnosis Suspicion

The Internet is a marvelous thing. Nowadays, anybody can look up medical information that was once the sole and private domain of doctors. This is both good and bad. The presence of the Internet has stripped away many of the medical profession's guarded secrets—exposing truths they had hoped nobody would ever discover. On the other hand, an excess of information—both facts and opinions can create mental unrest. The recently coined term, *cyberchondria* has been used to describe people who have caused themselves anxiety or even paranoia through self-diagnosis via Internet research. The word combines "cyber" for the Internet technology and "hypochondriac." A hypochondriac is a person who is excessively worried about developing an illness, or feels certain of having a particular disease—even though no medical evidence proves it so. A hypochondriac also tends to misinterpret every minor symptom (or even normal bodily functions) as symptoms of a serious illness.

The implication is that reading about symptoms and illness has a psychological effect, which can result in further symptoms. Once a person becomes focused on Lyme *Borrelia*, it becomes easy to view every bodily sensation (normal or abnormal) as being caused by it alone. This is simply not the case. In my opinion, focusing one's energy on Lyme disease is biggest obstacle towards achieving wellness. I understand that this may seem like a very strange statement to make in a book about Lyme disease! But hang in there—I promise you will fully understand what I mean once you have finished the upcoming chapter on diagnosis.

Is the Internet really making you ill? No, but I believe it is making you very *confused*. The symptoms associated with Lyme disease are so varied and complex. A web surfer can easily be lead down a path to pondering all kinds of diagnoses, syndromes, and conditions. An argument can be made that public accessibility to medical information can be hazardous to our health. Indeed, there are people making medical decisions on their own that would be best left up to competent doctors. However, in the case of Lyme disease, doctors have significantly let people down, leaving sick and suffering folks little choice but to do research on their own, as well as self-diagnose and self-treat.

Massive confusion and anxiety appear to result from all of the Internet chatter. It is ironic that a book as large this one needed to be written to explain and *simplify* the subject! The smokescreen had long been set to obstruct your view of your condition. Thanks to the Internet, I have had easy access to hundreds of research papers published in medical journals from around the world. With a few clicks, I can read about any virus, bacteria, or other microscopic life form—and their association to medical conditions. What have I learned? It turns out that scientists have known for a long time many causes of illnesses that it seems the public has been led to believe remain mysteries. It turns out that the same symptoms the Lyme community has come to associate with Lyme disease can equally be caused by hundreds, if not thousands of *other* microorganisms, chemicals, mechanical/neurological problem in the spine, and other factors. Therefore, going through a checklist of extremely common symptoms, and concluding "that sounds just like me," does not mean that tick-borne infection is the reason for every symptom.

Why are Doctors So Unwilling to Diagnose Lyme Disease?

Borrelia is merely one culprit among countless species of menacing microbes. It is not feasible for doctors to test for *hundreds* of different microorganisms that commonly trigger illness upon every patient encounter. Our already catastrophically high health care costs would rise exponentially. The Lyme Western Blot blood test is hardly the only medical test with questionable accuracy. Other infectious agents, as well as chemicals, and other causes can be equally problematic. What about all of the potential infections that are *not* bacterial? Is it practical or possible to test for every virus, protozoan, worm, and fungus?

Diagnosis of Inconvenience?

Perhaps it is medically *inconvenient* to pursue the diagnosis of tick-borne infection. Consider a healthy individual, who becomes ill after being bitten by a tick. One may logically suspect the symptoms are likely the result of Lyme and common co-infections. However, people commonly are unaware of being bitten by ticks, and many do not develop an expanding red rash. Over time, various symptoms develop— never considered as being triggered by tick-borne infection. Depending on what doctor, or type of doctor seen, the patient could be diagnosed and treated in a wide variety of ways. A family internist might diagnose the patient with Chronic Fatigue

Syndrome and express that no treatment or cure exists. A neurologist might diagnose the patient with peripheral neuropathy and prescribe drugs to try to mask the symptoms. The diagnosis of fibromyalgia might be issued by a rheumatologist, with the subsequent prescription of one of the aggressively-marketed FDA-approved drugs. If attempts to manage the symptoms are ineffective, a referral to a psychiatrist might result in the diagnosis of depression with an assortment of antidepressant drugs.

All of these very common diagnoses in this hypothetical scenario could be well-justified. Nevertheless it would be blatantly inaccurate to suggest that tick-borne infection mimicked the disorders. It caused them! How can mainstream medicine honestly say one moment that the cause of an illness is unknown in one instance, but then state that a particular infection mimics it? It is a weak and non-committal stance to take. Tick-borne and other infections can and do cause dozens of symptoms. Furthermore, many medical diagnoses are merely stating in Latin, what the patient describes in English:

__Patient__: *"I have pins and needles down my legs with numbness in my toes."*

<u>Doctor</u>: *"You have peripheral neuropathy."*

__Patient__: *"I have headaches only on my left side, behind my eye, and I feel dizzy, and I throw up."*

<u>Doctor</u>: *"You have Migraines."*

__Patient__: *"My whole body hurts… I can't sleep, I'm always tired, and I feel depressed.*

<u>Doctor</u>: *"You have fibromyalgia syndrome."*

These are common scenarios. The problem is that these diagnoses lack any *substance*. There is no recognition of CAUSE factors. This is shameful because all symptom have one or more causes. A diagnosis without at least one proposed cause factor associated with it is an incomplete diagnosis. How about: Lyme induced Migraines? *Borrelia*-triggered peripheral neuropathy? Could it be that medical diagnosis "truth in advertising" would be disruptive to the health care system? If fibromyalgia was recognized by the public as being directly (or even indirectly) triggered by Lyme disease, would that not affect public perception of FDA-approved "fibromyalgia" drugs? Would fibromyalgia patients be questioning their prescribing physicians about treating the underlying cause? The whole Lyme disease/blood tests/antibiotics circus would be taken to even greater heights!

"October of 2012 I had reached the end of my rope. I could barely function. I too had been diagnosed with fibromyalgia, then "chronic fatigue syndrome." Then no real idea of a diagnosis at all. It was all I could do just to get through the day. It was at that time I was finally diagnosed with Lyme disease. I was blessed to find Dr. Liebell. I began treatment there and my Lyme is gone! Lyme is so complicated, as it comes along with many co-infections. Dr. Liebell and his treatments saved my life. I was a skeptic, but I had been suffering so much, it was worth trying anything. Thankfully it worked."
    – Catherine H., Virginia Beach, VA

Is Lyme Disease *Really* the "Great Pretender?"

The apathetic dogma that Lyme disease mimics other medical conditions is grossly simplistic and fiendishly deceptive. There is no disputing microorganisms are agents of disease. A highly-functional immune system is capable of fighting off all kinds of pathogens and parasites. *Borrelia*, like many other infectious agents can directly cause and/or indirectly trigger a wide variety of medical conditions. One harmful microbe may weaken your

37

body, creating fertile soil for countless other microbes to flourish. From this, chronic illness can develop. This includes the triggering of autoimmune conditions. Each unique individual responds differently to each potential agent of disease.

Lyme is better characterized as a great *instigator*. Infection *causes* many diseases; it does not mimic or imitate them. The various diagnoses that people are given based upon their signs and symptoms are, for the most part, correct because they accurately fit the criteria for the conditions for which they are labeled. However, what they lack is are the elements of causes. I submit that most of the time, people are *not* misdiagnosed. This is of course, consistent with the conventional model of medical treatment of chronic conditions, which emphasizes masking of symptoms regardless of their causes.

The published medical academic literature reveals *Borrelia* is capable of affecting any system of the human body. Therefore it should be an integral consideration for *all* medical evaluations. Unfortunately, for as long as conventional Western medicine focuses on treating symptoms by mating each with a drug and ignoring cause factors, tick-borne infection will be rarely considered. It is much easier, convenient, and more lucrative to diagnose everything else. I propose we stop this mimic madness. Diagnoses of rheumatoid arthritis, lupus, peripheral neuralgia, and others are not wrong; they simply do not acknowledge causes. Multiple sclerosis is a stunning example. Here's why:

The term, **multiple sclerosis** simply means many hardened tissues—specifically degeneration of nerve tissue called the myelin sheath. The diagnosis of MS does not imply *any* specific cause, but rather only its effects. What many do not know is that papers published in medical journals that have pointed to bacteria (including *Borrelia*), viruses, and fungi as precipitating factors in multiple sclerosis. It seems that tick-borne infections are capable of triggering autoimmune reaction, which in the case of MS, results in nerve destruction (demyelination) and sclerotic lesions associated with it.

Is it Lyme Disease, Multiple Sclerosis, or BOTH?

Both multiple sclerosis and chronic Lyme disease are diagnoses that can be based upon clinical symptoms, history, and physical findings. Often a neurologist studies an MRI of the brain, which reveals lesions of the white matter. However, this is a finding that may be present in both conditions. Unlike the accepted signs and symptoms of MS, chronic Lyme victims may have joint and muscle pains. Multiple sclerosis is considered a disease of the brain, central nervous system, as well as the optic (eye) nerve. Both chronic Lyme and multiple sclerosis share damage to nerves of movement and sensation, as well as cognitive dysfunction, weakness, eye problems, and many others. It appears that Lyme affects more areas of the nervous system— that is, if we are trying to distinguish one from the other. I am not!

Unfortunately, it seems that doctors have been willing to blindly trust the negative Lyme blood tests as a ruling out factor, and stick to the general diagnosis of multiple sclerosis. This acceptance of a disease with legendary status as of being of unknown causes (an *urban* legend) is, in my opinion, a tragic mistake. There are numerous well-known medical conditions that result from chronic infection. Syphilis (spirochaete bacteria like *Borrelia*) can cause demyelination in some people, too. Viruses such as Epstein Barr, as well as poisons produced by molds (mycotoxins) have been implicated as causes of multiple sclerosis. I have personally seen patients diagnosed by other physicians with Amyotrophic lateral sclerosis (ALS, commonly called Lou Gehrig's disease), who without a doubt had an infectious tick bite as the cause. Does that mean Lyme disease mimics ALS, or that it can *cause* it?

39

One can have a genetic predisposition or weakness toward developing a particular condition, such as MS or ALS that others do not share. It seems plausible that those who are genetically prone to these neurological conditions may be those for whom it is triggered by tick-borne infection. How helpful it would be for doctors to be forthcoming and state that MS or ALS can be caused by Lyme disease. It seems ridiculous to sheepishly state Lyme disease mimics them.

Science has always existed on the border between ignorance and knowledge. When the mainstream accepts any knowledge, it is usually long after some individual or group has presented an idea. Since the days of Louis Pasteur, medicine has been aware of the effects of microorganisms on our health. Medical researchers do not seem too keen on blaming infection for the vast array of 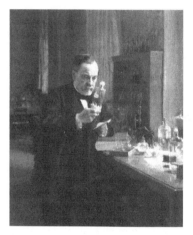 modern illnesses. It seems more dramatic, convenient, and tidy to give diseases fancy names—with little public attention to their various causes. In my opinion, it is patently ignorant to suggest Lyme mimics conditions such as multiple sclerosis, Parkinson's disease, fibromyalgia, or chronic fatigue syndrome. It is not if it is some outrageous idea to state that disease is spread by ticks, mosquitoes, flies, mites, fleas, and other biting critters. We know it is true. Medicine used to focus on microbes. Now it focuses on money-making drugs for conditions. The financial dilemma is that a great percentage of what ails people is viral in origin—and the drug treatment options are virtually nil. Still, it is important to understand that the bacterium of Lyme disease is but one small component of illness.

It is no great revelation that with chronic illness lies chronic infection. For conventional medical evaluation, it ought to always be a question of what organisms are affecting each patient. Could it be that most of us are exposed to *Borrelia* bacteria? I suspect it may be hard *not* to be. **Prior to an infectious tick bite, all victims *already* naturally harbor viruses, bacteria, fungi, protozoa (micro-parasites), and macro-parasites (helminth worms, insects, etc.). However, if a powerful enough force disturbs normal function of the victim's immune system, any existing germs can garner their forces for attack.** Another way of putting it is that a tick-borne infection can wreak havoc on an immune system that previously had viruses, bacteria, fungi, and other parasites under control—then it becomes "party time" for the microbes!

The One-Cause, One-Cure Catastrophe

Early Lyme disease can result in flu-like symptoms such as fever, chills, sweats, muscles aches, fatigue, nausea and joint pain. Some people develop Bell's palsy (paralysis of the facial nerve, which originates in the brain). Many agree that symptoms of chronic (late stage) or post-treatment Lyme disease syndrome (PTLDS) can include: headaches, neck problems, cognitive problems (memory, speech difficulties, etc.) increased sensitivity to light or sound, sleep disturbance, anxiety, depression, mood swings, fatigue, arthritis, abdominal pain, nausea, diarrhea, chest pain, palpitations, breathing problems, numbness, tingling or burning sensations (neuropathies). One must wonder, if all of these symptoms and syndromes can be caused by Lyme disease, why is there such controversy? Why isn't doxycycline heralded as the cure for all of the above? The answer is simple: all of these symptoms are commonly caused by non-bacterial sources too! We can visualize this with the analogy of a tree. Western medicine focuses on the leaves, but the roots are often ignored:

41

Are ALL Your Symptoms Caused by Lyme Disease?

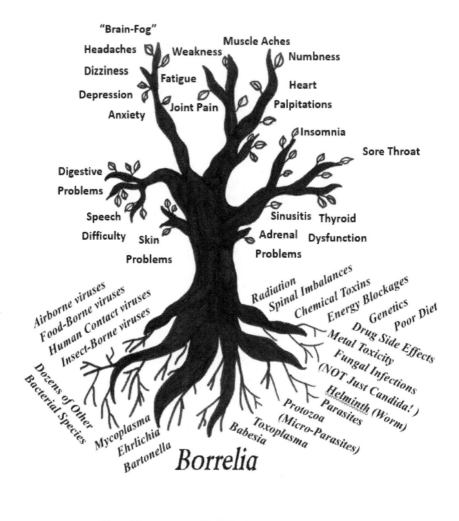

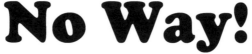

One of my patients, who was making progress under my care, after years of struggle, came to me feeling extremely puzzled. She said, "Dr. Liebell, why are doctors so afraid to diagnose Lyme disease?" I explained to her that many doctors simply don't know they're making a serious mistake when they carelessly rule out Lyme disease by negative blood tests. Published studies have shown them to be unreliable. Perhaps it's never occurred to them to study the subject. It is certainly possible that some doctors truly believe they have been thorough in ruling out Lyme, and move on to other less controversial or established diagnoses—medically accepted conditions like fibromyalgia, arthritis, migraines, peripheral neuropathy, MS, and dozens of others. That way, whatever popular medications are accepted for those conditions may be prescribed. Are they worried they'll look bad if someone figures out what's really wrong, and help people get well?" She replied. But I didn't answer her; I thought it was a *rhetorical question.*

She said, "I get it… but why can't they prescribe antibiotics for *suspected* cases of Lyme… they prescribe them for colds and all kinds of minor problems all the time?" This was a great question, and I explained that officially diagnosing Lyme is also a nuisance to physicians. There is annoying paperwork involved, plus it becomes ethically inappropriate to prescribe popular medications meant for other chronic and incurable conditions. So I asked her, what do you think would happen to the *business* of medicine if people stopped taking prescriptions for conditions actually triggered by *Lyme?* She understood. If a person gets diagnosed with fibromyalgia, one of the popular medicines could be prescribed indefinitely—to manage the symptoms of a supposedly incurable invisible disease, for which no cause is allegedly known. It would threaten profits if Lyme were diagnosed instead! My patient wanted me to try to help her understand the controversy over antibiotic usage for those who happen to be correctly diagnosed with Lyme. She cried, "How can the medical community believe antibiotics cure it, if so many people are still sick after taking them?" In the *business* of modern medicine, if the conventional establishment says "you're cured," it opens the doors to diagnose and treat other syndromes with highly profitable drugs.

They Can't Handle the Truth!"

Another patient of mine visited her rheumatologist (arthritis specialist). She had faithfully gone to this doctor for many years. She took many prescriptions to manage the symptoms associated with several different diagnoses, including lupus and fibromyalgia. At no time did this rheumatologist even mention Lyme disease. She bubbled with enthusiasm, telling the doctor how much she had improved over the last 6 months... until the doctor heard that it was due to *my* holistic wellness treatment!

She told the doctor that she no longer needed most of the medications he had prescribed her. She explained her revelation that her problems were triggered by tick-borne infection all those years ago, but now she was well. What do you think her doctor said? Was he thrilled at her drastic improvement? You'd like to think so, but, no. Did the doctor express his joy that she did not need the drugs anymore? Not by a long shot. Did he ask for my name and contact information, so he could learn more about the effects of tick-triggered illness, and the natural treatment that got her well? Dream on! The stony silence that settled between the woman and her doctor was painful. The specialist she trusted for years, and *believed* cared about her, threw down her file, spoke not a word, and promptly turned around and left the room with a slam of the door, and he never returned! She was discharged as a patient. Quite the "humanitarian," wasn't he?

Direct Diagnosis = Drug Dispersal

I have no doubt that if the public received an honest explanation of the bacterial cause of many medical conditions, it would incite a riot—an uncontrollable frenzy of antibiotic-seeking patients clamoring for the services of prescription-pushing physicians. The controversy of Lyme disease revolves around justification for long-term antibiotic treatment, and insurance companies to *pay for it*. That's right, I said it! Somebody had to say it! We can sugar coat this issue all we like, but it does not change reality. Why do you think so many people pay out-of-pocket for more blood tests? Their goal is to keep trying until they get a positive test—so a doctor can medically rationalize prescribing more antibiotics. They want proof of bacterial infection. The "battle cry" is for official medical proof to warrant insurance coverage for doxycycline and other drugs.

Medicine has a fascinating and a remarkable history of saving lives and healing the sick. Despite its mighty institutions, extraordinary scientific developments, and other magnificent achievements, we cannot assume that medical tests are infallible. We simply cannot trust blood tests for Lyme disease. In all fairness, there are all kinds of medical tests which are imperfect. I have made a career of helping people who were told there tests reveal "nothing is wrong." Diagnosis is far from a perfect science. A great deal of it is a matter of opinion, and many medical tests yield inconclusive, incorrect, or misleading results.

Medicine is nothing like it is depicted in the movies and television. Doctors cannot run tests for everything and get definitive answers. This is the harsh reality. With regards to Lyme disease, various ongoing investigations continue to confirm that it is not acceptable to solely rely on blood tests. Therefore, if a doctor tells you that Lyme disease has been ruled out by a Western Blot or ELISA Lyme blood test, you are not getting the full story.

Chapter 5

The Diagnosis You Dread...
"It's All in Your Head!"

It is unconscionable how frequently doctors tell patients, *"It's all in your head."* How egotistical, ignorant, incompetent, and lazy these so-called professionals are to assume a psychiatric condition merely because *they* cannot arrive at another diagnosis. Their pompous rationale is that once standard physical and laboratory tests, and diagnostic imaging come up empty—it must be a mental problem. Those who have suffered such indignity from these disgraceful professionals deserve a better fate.

The Inflamed Brain Doctors Just Won't Explain

Encephalitis is the medical term for swelling or inflammation of the brain. *Primary* encephalitis is defined as direct infection by an infectious organism. It can be the result of a recent illness, or an old one that is reactivating. There is a wealth of published medical research implicating various viral, protozoan, fungal, and bacterial infections. This of course includes *Borrelia*. One can even get an intestinal parasite through food that migrates to the brain. However, the diagnosis of encephalitis is typically restricted to extreme cases of acute infection. Standard tests for encephalitis include: MRI and CT-scan of the brain, evaluation of cerebro-spinal fluid (CSF) through lumbar spinal tap, virus DNA tests and other blood work, brain biopsy, and electroencephalogram (EEG).

Like many medical tests, negative results are not uncommon despite persistence of telltale symptoms. Victims of tick-triggered illness suffer a vast array of brain-related symptoms, which typically receive distinct diagnoses. This includes headaches, dizziness, ear noises (tinnitus), vision problems, light or sound hypersensitivity, memory problems, (often referred to as "brain fog"), seizures, and numerous psychiatric disorders! Ironically, this means there is a kernel of truth to the assertion of some of those contemptuous doctors who dismiss your problems as being "all in your head." Although they have no clue why, they are *sort of right*—but for the completely wrong reasons!

Turhan Canli, Ph.D., Associate Professor of Integrative Neuroscience at *Stony Brook University* recently argued that major depression results from infection, with likely genetic components (Source: *Reconceptualizing major depressive disorder as an infectious disease. Biology of Mood & Anxiety Disorders* 2014 4:10).

Head Games

Headaches are logically one of the symptoms of encephalitis. The pain is associated with the nerves, blood vessels, and muscles of your head and neck, as well as the membrane that covers your brain and spinal cord—the meninges. But what happens if there is no sign of acute infection—can headaches persist? Published medical research says unequivocally, YES. How this is addressed in clinical practice is another story. With over 8 million doctor visits per year, headaches are one of the most common medical complaints Americans have, costing tens of billions of dollars annually for medical management. Prescription headache medicines are a staple for many Lyme disease victims.

"After going undiagnosed with Lyme disease for over twelve years I finally found out I had a tick-borne disease. After being treated by my regular doctor with antibiotics, I didn't get any better and he didn't seem interested in figuring out another course of treatment. Found a "Lyme-literate doctor" and started getting more information about the disease and tried multiple courses of strong antibiotics. Unfortunately I just kept getting worse and worse. I didn't know where to turn and then my father-in-law learned of Dr. Liebell. His course of treatments have made me so much better. It has been such a long road. Not sure where I would be had it not been for Dr. Liebell." - Chris M. – Chincoteague, Virginia

Secondary or *post-infection* encephalitis is considered to be a disrupted immune system response that is triggered by infection in the brain that is no longer present. Much like other symptoms associated with tick-triggered illness, post-infection encephalitis is a scientifically verified phenomenon. Oddly, our government medical health institutions suggest that most people who have encephalitis have no symptoms, or perhaps a few mild ones. It is said that infectious causes of encephalitis cannot be determined in the *majority* of cases. How do they know this? How often are asymptomatic people tested for encephalitis? Of course it is very easy to find people who have some of these "mild" symptoms including: headaches, joint or muscle aches, fatigue, confusion, visual disturbances, and others. I feel certain that the vast majority of patients who seek my care suffer some degree of post-infection encephalitis.

Various common causes of encephalitis have been well-documented in medical journals:

Herpes Viruses, including *Varicella zoster* (Shingles), cytomegalovirus (CMV), and Epstein-Barr virus are examples. These viruses are notorious for going into hiding—remaining in the body long after the acute illness has faded away. These microbes have been implicated by scientists as causes of daily chronic headaches that are unresponsive to conventional treatment approaches.

48

Arborviruses are spread by insects and ticks (arthropods). They are usually named for the region where they were first discovered, such as the case with the West Nile virus. It is thought to have originated in Africa, but was discovered in New York in 1999, and is known to be present in most of the United States.

The presence of arboviruses are yet another reason why obsession with diagnosis of Lyme disease and antibiotic treatment is unproductive.

Enteroviruses are spread through food, water, and through the air by sneezing and coughing. Coxsackie virus, common cold, flu and other chest or throat viruses, as well as "stomach flu" viruses (Noroviruses, for example) can cause encephalitis.

Protozoan parasites (micro-parasites) and even parasitic worms (macro-parasites) can cause encephalitis. The Raccoon roundworm, *Baylisacaris procyonis* is an example. People can easily come in contact with it from soil, wood chips, and tree bark. This parasite apparently does not harm the raccoons, but it can impair the human nervous system, and certainly may cause encephalitis headaches.

Fungi, such as *Cryptococcus neoformans* can cause encephalitis, particularly in those who have poorly functioning immune systems.

Is Your Brain Feeling as "Dense as London Fog"?

"Brain fog" has become well-known jargon to describe confusion, forgetfulness, and difficulty concentrating. While technically not a medical term, nor recognized as a psychiatric diagnosis, brain fog solidly conveys meaning to experienced and understanding doctors. Many who are bitten by infectious ticks develop these symptoms, yet diagnostic tests (MRI, CT scans, neurological tests, blood tests, etc.) reveal no abnormalities. The wide variety of microbes that can cause encephalitis may be causes for altered mental clarity. Brain fog is not exclusive to Lyme disease. Toxins, nutritional problems, and even structural imbalances can contribute to brain fog.

It is my assertion that a tremendous number of sufferers of headaches, dizziness, vision problems, and brain fog are living lives of misery because of undetected encephalitis. The standard tests neither reveal discernible brain inflammation, nor do they detect acute infection. Yet the symptoms persist. So much for modern technology! As you will learn in later chapters, in the field of energy medicine, we understand that we can gain further insight into human health by observing the subtle electromagnetic energies of the body, when chemical and physical medical evaluations come up empty.

Morgellons Mistreatment Mania

The unfortunate folks who suffer from Morgellons disease are certain that worms or bugs of some kind are crawling under the skin. It certainly looks and feels like this is the case. However, victims of this malady are horrendously treated as *psychiatric* cases because no bugs, worms, or microbes are found under the skin. Who are the crazy ones? No doubt it's the arrogant and ignorant doctors who clearly see a wretched skin problem, but tell the patient it's a delusional disease! Fortunately, Morgellons sufferers were vindicated by a 2018 medical study providing proof it is REAL; it is the abnormal production of fibrous protein filaments in the skin triggered by spirochetal infection.

Source: Middelveen MJ, Fesler MC, Stricker RB. History of Morgellons disease: from delusion to definition. *Clinical, cosmetic and investigational dermatology*. 2018;11:71-90.

"The nervous system is the principal target for a number of metals. Inorganic compounds of aluminum, arsenic, lead, lithium, manganese, mercury, and thallium are well known for their neurological and behavioral effects in humans" - Clarkson TW. Metal toxicity in the central nervous system. *Environmental Health Perspectives.* 1987;75:59-64.

Chapter 6

Metallic Misdiagnosis Mayhem

Heavy metal toxicity is the result of excessive accumulation of certain metals in the body. It can contribute to the development of a great diversity of serious chronic medical conditions, although seemingly scarcely considered in most clinical medical practice. The function of hundreds of hormones and trillions of biochemical functions of the body can be impaired by metal toxicity. This includes interference with normal balance and location of nutritional minerals in the body. It is no wonder why many nutritional approaches fail. It is not a question of lack of dietary nutrients, but rather compromised utilization of them within the body.

Metals can accumulate and affect the function of your brain, liver, heart, bones, and other organs. They are thought to potentially affect your DNA, which has been linked with cancer. Our conventional medical establishment acknowledges that acute toxicity can result from high levels of metals in your body. Regrettably, it seems massive numbers of people suffer the ill effects of chronic low-level accumulation. Heavy metals are everywhere, and exposure cannot be entirely avoided. As is the case with nearly any cause of illness, there may be a genetic predisposition for some to suffer metal detoxification difficulties. Those afflicted by tick-triggered illness seem to clearly become inefficient at eliminating them through the body's normal detoxification and drainage pathways.

Aluminum Alert

The list of possible symptoms related to aluminum toxicity is staggering! It may contribute to, or directly cause: Alzheimer's disease, confusion, dementia, Parkinson's disease, behavioral problems, learning disabilities, colds, gastrointestinal problems, low energy, distorted immune function, restless legs, liver problems, kidney problems, headaches, heartburn/reflux, numbness, osteoporosis, skin problems, and muscle aches.

How does aluminum get into your body? It is frightening how many sources of toxic aluminum exist. Just a few of them include: antiperspirants and deodorants, cookware, dental amalgams, tobacco smoke, toothpastes, water supply, many pharmaceutical medicines, dust, wiring, ceramics, baking powder, beer, auto exhaust, aluminum foil and cans, cosmetics, and pesticides.

Loaded with Lead

We are pelted with lead from many sources. It can come from cigarette smoke, inks, pesticides, children's toys, city water, paint, pottery, cosmetics, household dust, auto exhaust, canned fruit and juice, and various other industrial sources. Lead toxicity can cause abdominal pains, adrenal gland dysfunction, kidney problems, peripheral neuropathies, numbness, joint pain, insomnia, headaches, depression, attention deficit disorder, allergies, anxiety, muscle weakness, thyroid problems, memory loss, menstrual problems, fatigue, and many other symptoms.

Cadmium Catastrophe

Cadmium toxicity has a shockingly long list of potential symptoms associated with it, including infertility, flu-like symptoms, bone disease, migraines, osteoporosis, liver damage, alopecia (hair loss disease), impotence, digestive difficulties, kidney disease, and many others. If you are a smoker, you are inhaling cadmium every day. Not only is cadmium found in cigarette smoke, but also in some sodas, refined grains and cereals, fish, tap water, and various environmental and industrial contaminants.

Mercury Madness

If you suffer chronic fatigue, perhaps it is not all due to tick-triggered illness or Epstein-Barr virus. Mercury toxicity can cause adrenal glands dysfunction, in addition to a mind-blowing number of symptoms including: speech disorders, nerve degeneration, thyroid dysfunction, memory loss, skin problems, suicidal tendencies, joint pain, migraines, dizziness, hyperactivity, depression, loss of coordination, vision problems, and hearing loss.

Mercury sources are numerous, including all kinds of manufacturing and industrial production. Mercury is, of course, found in some dental fillings. Many patients have presented to me having already had holistic dentist remove them, as part of their quest for recovery. I rarely, if ever suggest this to be done, although I am not against it in some cases. In general, it is not the mercury from dental fillings that is my concern, but rather the body's struggle to eliminate incoming sources from cosmetics, fabric softeners, seafood, tattoos, laxatives, pesticides, and yes—our water supply. Mercury can "light the fire" to many chronic illnesses, and seems to be a major factor with tick-triggered illness. It is one of the most poisonous metals on the planet.

Copper Conundrum

If you're suffering depression, copper toxicity could be a factor. The same is the case for yet another horrifying long list of symptoms, including: allergies, fatigue, thyroid dysfunction, insomnia, decreased sex drive, panic attacks, urinary tract infections, yeast infections, mood swings, and many more. Copper toxicity, like *Borrelia* has also been linked with multiple sclerosis. Copper can get into your body from cookware, dental fillings, pesticides, industrial emissions, birth control pills, beer, fish, chocolate, and many other food and industrial sources.

How Do We Protect Ourselves?
Is Intravenous Chelation Therapy the Solution?

Chelation therapy is not a part of the *Bio-energetic Individual Treatment Equation.*© This treatment is intended to suck up or bind (chelate) metals for the body to excrete. Insurance does not pay for it, and it costs $3,000 to $4,000 for a long series of treatments where you sit with an intravenous needle for 2-3 hours. However, its costs and inconvenience are not my objections. **The major drawback is that chelation does not change physiology**. In other words, even if you can suck out metals, the problem there is that the metals will likely keep coming back and accumulating—unless your body systems that are supposed to naturally eliminate them restore normal function. Forcing them out is temporary. Those who suffer poorly-functioning immune systems seem to lack full capacity to naturally eliminate metals. By the way, "naturally" does *not* mean forcing toxins out with an herbal cleanse or eating bushels of chlorella! It means your body is naturally doing it on its own. There's a big difference! For those who like the taste of cilantro, it is indeed a great food for supporting metal detoxification.

Core BITE Principle: What else do you think can impair your body's ability to eliminate toxic metals? That's right...antibiotics! Ironic it is that the standard treatment for Lyme disease could cause the same symptoms by creating a *different problem.*

Awareness of these toxins is a start. I recommend taking measures to reduce household sources of metal toxicity. But we cannot live in a "bubble." My three children attend public schools, and are exposed to various toxins (including molds and mildew) both there and in the outside world. My family is very careful about the foods we eat, the cleaning products we use, and various other measures. Can it be helpful to eat foods like cilantro, which have a metal detoxification effect? Of course. However, my experience has been that the most important step is bio-energetic supplement support, which will be explained in the treatment chapters ahead. When my wife Sheila had Lyme disease, homeopathic type detoxification of heavy metals was a critical factor in her complete recovery.

"The weakening of the immune system creates as a result changes in the physical body which we call pathology" - Dr. Samuel Hahnemann

Chapter 7

Microbes without Medicine:

The "Dirty Little Secret" that Keeps Victims of Tick-Borne Illness Sick

An antibiotic-centered approach to recovery completely misses three major types of microorganisms. In this chapter you will discover what *else* is making you sick, and why antibiotics can *never* help.

Going Viral

Viruses, like other non-bacterial pathogens cannot be killed by antibiotics. Why don't we have drugs to kill viruses? Viruses are protected from drugs because they reside *inside* human cells. The few antiviral medicines that do exist merely help keep viruses in check. Doctors are sternly warned by government health authorities to *never* treat viral illness with antibiotics. I shudder at how often this axiom of medicine is violated in daily practice with prescriptions being written for symptoms of colds and assorted infections for which no actual testing is performed—"just in case."

It is my view that a high percentage of symptoms tick-triggered illness sufferers experience are due to viruses. It could certainly be the case that initial tick-borne infection disrupts function of the immune system—leaving it more susceptible to numerous viruses, many of which resided in the body prior to the bite. It seems likely that many of the persistent symptoms associated with Lyme disease that remain after substantial antibiotic therapy are caused by viruses—microbes for which there is no medicine capable of killing. As we saw in the section on encephalitis, there are numerous types of tick and insect-borne, airborne, food and water-borne, and human contact viruses. Humans are constantly infected by viruses, but most of the time no symptoms are felt. Viruses can cause diseases ranging from colds to cancer.

Chronic Fatigue Syndrome was once a very popular diagnosis, for the symptoms likely triggered by the Epstein-Barr virus (EBV), which is associated with infectious mononucleosis ("mono"). However, there are no prescription medications to kill viruses. The *Centers for Disease Control* have reported on their website (CDC.gov) that as many as "95% of adults between 35 and 40 years of age have been infected." They also state that EBV is indistinguishable from other childhood illnesses. It has also been implicated in several autoimmune diseases, as well as some forms of cancer! **In my experience, many of the symptoms from which Lyme disease-obsessed patients suffer are caused by EBV and numerous other types of viruses, rather than exclusively *Borrelia*.**

Fungal in the Jungle

Cliché as it may be to say, there is toxic fungus among us. Fungi include mushrooms, yeast, molds and mildews. They do not get adequate medical and media attention—bacteria and viruses steal all the limelight. However, the presence of fungi in our environment and our bodies is nothing to take lightly. Recent research has proven that fungal toxins are responsible for way more human suffering than previously thought. Various health

57

problems may have fungi as one of their underlying causes, and it appears to be a major factor for those suffering from chronic tick-triggered illness.

Sadly, most conventional doctors seem to dismiss the significance of fungi. Lyme disease savvy professionals tend to be more aware. I have read numerous criticisms that the health threat of fungi is an exaggerated claim from practitioners of alternative medicine. Those naive individuals, who hold such an opinion should be mortified by their own ignorance, and hang their heads in shame! I pity their patients, since medical journals contain a mountain of evidence that supports fungi as a significant health threat!

While some fungi, such as mushrooms can be food—many fungi are *germs*. Some fungi can even be deadly. They can infect your skin, nails or hair (dermatomycosis). An example is *Tinea* or ringworm. It gets its name because it looks like worms under the skin (but it's actually a fungus!). I have even seen cases of Lyme disease that were misdiagnosed as ringworm! Athlete's foot and Jock Itch are also examples of fungal problems. Fortunately, these surface infections can usually be treated effectively by medication, and it doesn't often spread to internal organs. Other fungal problems are more troublesome.

Candida is species of fungus that grows in soft and moist areas of the body. Candida overgrowth, like other fungal infections may result from antibiotic treatment. This can happen because the medicine that kills the harmful bacteria also kills off the beneficial bacteria. The helpful bacteria would normally compete with the yeast, but when killed off, enables the yeast free to grow too much. This results in a yeast infection. If you have taken lots of antibiotics, you surely have fungal concerns. In my opinion, merely taking probiotic supplements will unlikely make a dent in the fungal frenzy!

Fungi can also affect your nervous system or internal organs such as your lungs. Most fungal infections develop much more slowly, compared to those caused by bacteria. A fungal infection (called a mycosis) also tends to come back more often. In addition, your body does not develop lasting immunity to fungal infections as it can for bacterial. More serious fungal infections can affect your entire body (systemic mycosis).

Fungal spores (the reproductive seeds) can get into your body through openings in your skin. Soil can be infected with a spreadable fungus. Fungal spores may be breathed in through the air, contributing to various respiratory diseases. Coccidiomycosis is a fungal infection caused by a form of yeast that attaches to dust, which is breathed in. Such a fungal infection can cause symptoms that seem identical to flu! *Cryptococcus* can cause encephalitis, particularly in those who have dysfunctional immune systems. There are more than 30 species of these fungi. Clearly, fungal woes go far beyond *Candida*—the fungus that gets most of the public attention.

Poisonous substances emitted by fungi are called mycotoxins. They commonly reside in contaminated fruits, vegetables, cereals, and nuts. *Aspergillus* is an example of a fungus that produces mycotoxins, which can be spread to people. Farm animals that eat fungus-contaminated grain can transmit mycotoxins to people through their meat or milk. This *Aspergillus*-produced poison, specifically called aflatoxin is a powerful cancer-causing agent. Mycotoxins can damage your lymphatic system, including your bone marrow. Scientists are now confirming that more problems are caused by fungi than ever considered.

A 1999 Mayo Clinic study revealed that an immune system response to several species of fungi is the cause of most chronic sinus infections! Prior to the release of this study, the cause was unknown. Tens of millions of Americans suffer from chronic sinusitis. The Mayo Clinic noted that fungus allergy was thought to be the cause of fewer than ten percent of cases. However, their studies showed that *fungi* are likely the cause of nearly all of these problems. They concluded that it is not an allergic reaction, but rather an immune reaction. What's the difference? Generally, an allergic reaction is when the body reacts abnormally to a substance that is otherwise harmless. It is normal and healthy for one's immune system to try to fight off a toxic fungus. However chronic sinusitis occurs when the immune system is NOT functioning adequately to win the ongoing battle with the fungi. The ongoing immune response irritates the sinuses in the process.

According to the *National Ambulatory Medical Care Survey* (2009), nearly 30 million Americans are diagnosed with sinusitis, with nearly 12 million diagnosed as chronic. Nearly $6 billion is spent in annual health care costs related to treatment! Isn't it time to accept that conventional Western medicine has massively bungled diagnosis and treatment of chronic sinusitis? It is frightening to know about this repulsive amount of hard-earned money that Americans are spending on sinusitis. Here is yet another example of the disastrous misuse of antibiotics. Lyme disease is hardly the only problem. 1999 was a long time ago. Despite this groundbreaking research being published by the world-famous Mayo Clinic, the way most doctors treat patients with chronic sinusitis does not to appear to have changed. Doctors are still writing antibiotics prescriptions for chronic sinus infections, despite the compelling scientific evidence refuting the value of antibiotic treatment for fungal infections.

One might wonder, why is anti-fungal treatment not a major focus in pharmaceutical research? The answer seems to lie in the fact that anti-fungal drugs have been found to be extremely risky. Their serious and even deadly side effects cannot be justified for potential benefits. Anti-fungal drugs pose serious risks of liver damage, allergic reactions, hormonal imbalances, and death. Fungal cells are nothing like bacteria cells, which can be killed by antibiotics. Drug companies have struggled to create safe and effective anti-fungal medicines because fungal cells are similar to *human* cells on the molecular level. Because of the similarities in biochemistry, anti-fungal drugs can harm human cells too. This is why doctors who practice holistic and natural methods have been desperately trying to get the medical establishment and the general public to understand the value of their treatments. There are various approaches used worldwide, which can support regulation of the body's natural ability to fight off germs, including fungi. One's immune system must deal with fungi to assure progressive and lasting improvement. You will learn in the later chapters how we support the body's natural fungus-fighting systems with the *Bio-energetic Individual Treatment Equation.*

The Protozoan Parasitic Puzzle

The term, parasite is one that generates much confusion for both doctors and patients. It is time to clear this up. A **parasite** is simply any organism that resides in (or on) another organism (the host)—causing some harm to it. Approximately one half of all existing animal species on earth are parasites! There are single-celled microscopic parasites **(micro-parasites)** and multi-celled larger ones **(macro-parasites)**. The term, **pathogen** is used typically reserved for micro-parasites, which include some species of bacteria, fungi, and protozoa, as well as viruses. Macro-parasites include **helminths**—tapeworms, flukes, and roundworms. They are transmitted primarily by feces-contaminated soil that contains their eggs. Many arthropods (bugs) are also macro-parasites. This includes ticks, mites, lice, fleas, and more than 100,000 different species of insects. These animals seek the blood of another animal.

The types of parasites to which most Lyme victims and their doctors refer are the protozoa and helminth worms. **Protozoa** are among the 10,000 different species of single-celled life forms. Protozoa can have characteristics of animal, plant, and fungal cells, but they are not similar to bacteria. Examples of protozoa include: *Blastocystis hominis, Giardia lambia, Toxoplasma gondii, Entamoeba histolytica, Babesia microti, Trypanosoma cruzi, Plasmodium falciparum, and Cryptosporidium*. People with poorly functioning immune systems tend to be at greater risk for suffering the effects of protozoan infection.

More Mind Games

You have already learned that a link between Lyme disease and mental illness has been established. It is hardly a new discovery that microorganisms can harm the human brain. Syphilis, which is caused by *Treponema pallidum*, a spirochaete bacteria (similar to *Borrelia*) has been long-known to trigger psychosis. Associations have been made by scientists between *Streptococcus* bacteria and obsessive compulsive disorder (OCD) and nervous tics such as in Tourette syndrome. The diagnosis of PANDAS (Pediatric Autoimmune Neuropsychiatric Disorders Associated with Streptococcal Infections) has been recently conceived for this. Research has also shown a relationship between a herpes virus and bipolar disorder.

The Crazy Cat Calamity

Further evidence that mental illness has parasitic causes in the brain is **Toxoplasma gondii**. Like its cousins *Babesia* and *Plasmodium* (Malaria), *Toxoplasma* is a protozoan. It is one of the most common infectious microorganisms in the world. It is a parasite that has been reported in medical literature to be significant in people whose immune systems are severely impaired, particularly in the case of AIDS. Common symptoms associated with *Toxoplasma* include headache, confusion, seizures, coordination problems, and fever. According to the *Centers for Disease Control* (CDC.gov), Toxoplasmosis is considered to be a leading cause of death attributed to food borne illness in the United States. It has been suggested that *Toxoplasma* can result in impairment in reaction time, which can in turn, increase one's chances of auto accidents. It has been linked with anti-social, aggressive, and jealous behavior in men, as well as promiscuity in women. The implication is that it can affect one's thoughts and actions.

Toxoplasma is commonly spread through handling or eating undercooked and contaminated meat, such as lamb, pork, or venison. However, this microbe reproduces primarily inside cats. The cats get infected from eating infected mice, rats, birds, and other small animals, and spread *Toxoplasma* through their feces. This is why pregnant women are advised to never clean cat litter boxes. Outdoor cats can contaminate water and soil with *Toxoplasma*, thus one does not need to have direct contact with a cat, or infected meat to have this microbe enter the body. Poultry livestock that are fed *Toxoplasma*- contaminated food or water can become infected. Unwashed fruits or vegetables can even spread it, which is why I suggest avoid eating *uncooked* foods from restaurants (that's right… salads can be bad for you!).

Does this mean cats could be making you crazy? It is quite possible. The CDC states that more than 60 million Americans carry the *Toxoplasma* parasite, and frankly admit it is a neglected parasitic infection! According to the *U.S. Department of Health and Human Services - National Institutes of health* (www.niaid.nih.gov), very few medicines can fight protozoa, and some of those are either harmful to humans or are becoming ineffective. The drugs could actually harm a person more than the parasite does. Even if there were *safe* medications that could kill parasites, obliterating every one of them would be absolutely impossible. There are too many species, which would require too many drugs. I find dubious the claim that the combination of black walnut hulls, Wormwood (from the Artemisia shrub), and cloves will kill most of your helminth parasites. I consistently encounter patients who have failed to respond to this and other parasite cleanses.

Our government health authorities profess that a *strong immune system* is how one best deals with *Toxoplasma*, since there is no medical cure. This is indeed where holistic wellness-based health care must come to the rescue. Once again, we have a microbe that can get into our brains that cannot be killed by antibiotics. Antibiotics kill bacteria. They are ineffective against most other infectious microbes including viruses, fungi, and protozoa, which massively combine forces as agents of disease. They are microbes for which there is no medicine.

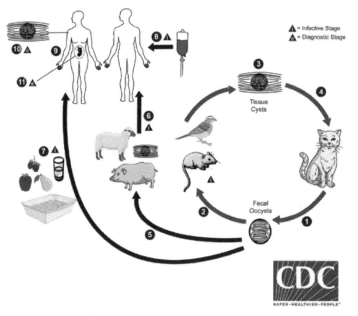

Source: www.cdc.gov/dpdx/toxoplasmosis/index.html

Chapter 8

Adrenal Fatigue

Do you have a hard time getting up in the morning? Do you need coffee, or caffeinated sodas to rev yourself up upon awakening, or to pep up during the day? Are you struggling to cope with stress? Has your desire for sex decreased? If the answer is "yes" to any of these questions, it is likely that you are suffering from the effects of adrenal gland dysfunction. It may also be called adrenal fatigue, burnout, or exhaustion. Located above your kidneys are the adrenal glands. These are glands that are critical to your health and wellbeing. The adrenal glands secrete the hormones that help your body deal with stress and regulate many bodily functions. They respond to the input from your nervous system. "Burnout" is when the functional ability of your adrenal glands is low. It is not simply fatigue, which can be handled by a few decent nights of sleep. It is better described as profound exhaustion of your body's energy-making systems. Fatigue is merely one symptom. You might actually sleep well, but your body is not energized by sleep.

What Causes Adrenal Exhaustion?

Common causes include chronic infection, emotional stress, chemical and electromagnetic toxicity, structural imbalances, poor nutrition, and energetic blockages. Working too hard, stressful family problems and too much mental stimulation are huge factors in harming the adrenal glands. Our lives are loaded with fear and stress. It's no wonder people are such a mess. We are all exposed to endless supply of harmful chemicals. If you are healthy, your body is better equipped to get rid of these toxins. Toxic buildup makes your adrenal glands weaker.

Another giant factor is the stress of harmful electromagnetic fields. Such fields generated by cell phones, microwave ovens, power lines, and computers, etc. are easily dismissed, but can significantly threaten our health. Poor nutrition may seem obvious, but there's more to it than just taking an extra multivitamin. When your stress is high, your adrenal glands need *better* nutrition. This includes clean water and naturally occurring minerals. You can even have nutritional deficiencies passed down to you from your mother during pregnancy. This is not genetics, but rather fetal development. A child can be born already at a disadvantage if the mother is nutritionally deficient and in a state of adrenal exhaustion.

Stimulants Damage Your Adrenal Glands

The boost that you might be getting from your daily coffee, cola drink, or caffeinated tea is damaging your adrenal glands and contributing to chronic fatigue and pain. Sugar, caffeine and alcohol are devastating to your adrenals. Too much or too intense exercise can even contribute. While it may feel good short-term, excessive exercise can have a negative effect on the adrenals. I advise most of my patients to stop vigorous exercise for a while, unless an individual thoroughly convinces me it is beneficial. This gives the adrenal glands a fighting chance to recover.

Emotional Causes

Your emotions, particularly rage, hatred and anger play an important role. Taking control of the emotional component is a critical factor in overcoming adrenal exhaustion. Becoming able to deal better with stress is a critical factor in overcoming adrenal exhaustion. Many emotional and psychological symptoms can be present with adrenal exhaustion. If you feel apathy, hopelessness, despair, irritability, anxiety, anger, resentment, or feel a loss of faith in people, you could be suffering from adrenal exhaustion.

66

Other Symptoms

Low blood pressure, blood sugar, or body temperature, are common symptoms. Food and chemical sensitivities and allergies may result from adrenal burnout, as a result of low levels of the hormone, cortisol. Thyroid imbalances can develop as a result of adrenal burnout. The thyroid and adrenal glands share a close relationship, thus a problem in one affects the other. When your adrenals are weak, you are susceptible to toxic buildup of copper. This negatively affects your emotions. When your energy is low, your body loses its ability to eliminate toxic metals, which also can cause countless physical and psychological symptoms. Other common symptoms include depression, joint pain, back pain, as well as craving for salt and sugar. Notice that these are symptoms commonly attributed to Lyme disease!

Core Biting Back Principle: Understanding the multiple causes and effects of adrenal dysfunction helps you understand why you must not obsess with or blame any single microorganism infection as the sole cause of your symptoms. Active Lyme *Borrelia* infection may be long gone, but its cascading effects can remain.

Symptoms from adrenal dysfunction may not rise to the surface for many years after a causative event. Unfortunately, most physicians do not acknowledge adrenal fatigue. Millions of prescriptions for antidepressant drugs and sleep medicine are testimony to this. Adrenal dysfunction is often dismissed as an alternative medicine phenomenon. Perhaps this is because it is not a condition for which a prescription drug can be marketed. There is no billable medical diagnosis insurance code either. Unless one is diagnosed with Addison's disease, a very severe form adrenal dysfunction, adrenal dysfunction is rarely considered. Conventional laboratory testing typically does not reveal evidence of adrenal deficiency. It is more of a clinical conclusion made by holistic-minded practitioners who understand that health is much more than blood test results being within normal ranges.

Although adrenal dysfunction is a biochemical problem, it can affect you emotionally. In my opinion, it must be taken seriously and naturally treated, as a primary approach. People are laboring through their lives with adrenal burnout. They are so busy that they don't realize how exhausted their bodies actually are. Many people appear to be healthy, but they are actually highly stressed.

We live in a quick fix health care society. However, there are absolutely no shortcuts to recovery from adrenal fatigue. It takes time and energy. It is like rebuilding your body from scratch. It's not a minor repair. It can take a year or two to fully recover, so it requires a serious commitment to your health. Is this a long time? Having a baby takes nine months, and orthodontic braces may be needed for several years to straighten out crooked teeth. Although it absolutely can be done, naturally restoring adrenal function is no small feat. For example, some patients overcome serious chronic pain and cognitive problems they associated with Lyme disease within six months. However, it takes them much longer to feel energetic again. Others restore energy rapidly, but require more healing time to resolve pain and other symptoms.

I advise my patients to avoid stimulants and chemicals that mask symptoms—creating an illusion of energy and well-being. Improper adrenal function can lead to other degenerative diseases and must be taken very seriously if you really want to get healthy again. You may find that the people in your life do not understand all of the challenges of recovery. Adrenal fatigue can contribute to damaged relationships. It is a complex and demanding problem to overcome, but tremendously rewarding once properly evaluated and treated.

Core Biting Back Principle: Facilitating recovery from adrenal fatigue is a critical component of the BITE for most patients. But you cannot simply take adrenal supplements to enable repair. Your immune system must FIRST function better to combat the chronic infection and toxicity that typically <u>causes</u> the adrenal fatigue! Although a diet rich in nutritious whole foods is advisable, it may be minimally effective as long as the adrenal glands continue to be assaulted.

"The trouble with the world is not that people know too little; it's that they know so many things that just aren't so."

- Mark Twain

Part Three:

Myths, Misconceptions, and Mistakes:

What NOT to Do (and Why)

Discover Why Preconceived Notions about Lyme Disease, and Limiting Beliefs about Your Health Can Hold You Back From the Life You Deserve

"If I could live my life over again, I would devote it to proving that germs seek their natural habitat: diseased tissue—rather than being the cause of diseased tissue—ex: mosquitoes seek stagnant water, but do not cause the pool to become stagnant." - Rudolf Virchow (1821-1902)

Chapter 9

Drug Obsessions and Prescription Confessions—Why Antibiotics May <u>Not</u> Be the Answer!

Mainstream medicine has conditioned Americans to expect restoration of health through treating infections with antibiotics. True health does not come from quick fix medicine, which gives little thought toward long term benefit. Consider the words of Dr. Virchow, the father of modern pathology, quoted above. You might be tempted to skip this chapter—especially if you are already fed up with the antibiotic approach to chronic Lyme disease. But please, do not skip it; you will miss out on critical information that will help you better understand your potential solution!

Here's why:

Did you know that only a *minority* of species of bacteria are capable of causing disease in humans? It is an undisputed scientific fact that antibiotics kill the beneficial bacteria that are vital to many functions of your body. Killing the good ones can leave you even more susceptible to the antibiotic resistant bacteria like MRSA (*Staphylococcus*), C. diff (*Clostridium difficile*), Anthrax, *Klebsiella pneumonia*, and many others. "Superbugs" as they are called. Antibiotics should be used *correctly*, so that when they are needed to save your life, they are effective! According to the CDC, Antibiotic resistance is one of the world's most

71

pressing public health problems. On their website, www.cdc.gov they state that most types of bacteria have become stronger and less responsive to antibiotic treatment when it is really needed. Are Lyme savvy doctors turning a blind eye to this fact?

The key to protecting yourself against antibiotic-resistant "superbugs" is to strengthen your body so these harmful life forms cannot survive and thrive inside you. This is the core principle of the *Bio-energetic Individual Treatment Equation.*© A dysfunctional immune system leaves you prey to numerous harmful things, including: antibiotic-resistant bacteria, viruses, fungi (not just Candida yeast), and other parasites that are transmitted through our food and water supply, the air, and from physical contact. Disturbances to normal immune system regulation often results in newly-developed food allergies and sensitivities to chemicals.

One of the most important steps you can take in your successful journey to recover from tick-triggered illness is accepting and understanding that your real problem is <u>damage to function and regulation of your immune system</u>. The solution is to support restoration of its normal and healthy self-regulation. Yes, *Borrelia* infection may have triggered the process and single-handedly caused damage—but it alone is unlikely the reason for all of the misery inflicted upon you. Most importantly, if your immune system does not make a legitimate comeback, you will not really be better. I remind you of what else contributes mightily to further damaging your immune system: antibiotics! They were never meant for long-term usage. As the *Centers for Disease Control* state (at www.cdc.gov), *"Repeated and improper uses of antibiotics are primary causes of the increase in drug-resistant bacteria."*

There is no disputing that antibiotics can be lifesaving; they are one of the greatest medical developments in history. That is not the issue here. We are talking about how repeated usage for suspected *Borrelia* infection will kill the beneficial bacteria in your body, and make it even harder for your body to handle the very germs it needs to eradicate!

Antibiotics have indeed been wonder drugs that have saved countless lives, and have served admirably in all kinds of emergencies. Their massive overuse and misuse has spoiled the party. Despite the warnings of top scientists that killing the beneficial bacteria along with the harmful species has dire consequences, the prescriptions persist prolifically. Overuse of antibiotics drives up health care costs dramatically.

I respect the long-term antibiotic-prescribing doctors' willingness to acknowledge Lyme disease. They deserve the benefit of the doubt of having nothing but good intentions. I am sincerely happy for those fortunate people who have responded to antibiotics (or any other method), and have stayed well. This book and its recommendations are not for those people, but rather the suffering souls for whom it has failed. It is of course also for those who do not want to take the antibiotic route in the first place.

The bottom line is one cannot promote life by *killing*. Antibiotics are designed for bacterial genocide. If only the entire kingdom of bacteria were our enemy. It is not. Most bacteria in our bodies are helpful and necessary, if not at least harmless. More collateral damage results from overuse and inappropriate use of the drugs than would have ever been considered, tracing back to the dawn of the antibiotic era. The realization of antibiotic resistant bacteria is not new, nor is it challenged medically. Nevertheless, mainstream medicine is still clinging to a militaristic view—a war against bacteria, demonstrated by its single-minded philosophy of antibiotic treatment for Lyme, and any other microbes that stand in its way (with or without proof of infection).

Patients consistently report their exasperation and devastation from being kept on antibiotics for years. Enthusiasm for the drugs eludes me, as new patients lament how their wallets were drained by the thousands (often tens of thousands) of dollars spent on LLMD visits, oral antibiotics, and PICC lines (Peripherally Inserted Central Catheter) for intravenous antibiotics… leaving them either no better or worse than before. Antibiotics are being administered at dosages and frequency far beyond medically valid standards of safety and effectiveness. Add to this the anti-microbial herbs prescribed to give the appearance of natural or holistic treatment.

Let's get this straight:

Antibiotics do not make your body stronger—they <u>weaken</u> your immune system. They do <u>not</u> kill the majority of parasites and pathogens. This is a long-established and undisputed scientific fact. The *National Institutes of Health* (NIH) research concluded that long term antibiotics are dangerous. Perhaps some doctors and patients believe they are their only hope. The controversies of Lyme are issues of money, greed, politics, and ignorance. Consider that there is hardly a shortage of antibiotic consumption in America. The NIH has not campaigned against their general usage. Nor have any other medical institutions. Antibiotics are one of the top selling products in medicine! So why would there be any objection or controversy associated with antibiotic usage for Lyme disease? Could it be because they really don't work in the manner for which they're claimed? Or is it because antibiotics are much less profitable than drugs designated for chronic neurological, heart, psychiatric, and arthritic conditions? How about the fact that most intelligent doctors *agree* that it is foolish to keep people on them when no active infection is confirmed?

This is another solid reason why the wellness model of health care is essential for those who are drowning in a sea of medical confusion and controversy. Holistic medicine is desperately needed—to provide effective treatment that does not depend on agreement over diagnostic standards, and poses no risk of bodily harm. What a relief and a thrill it has been for patients to receive highly-effective care—devoid of any controversy whatsoever. I do not share the fundamental assumption that success can only come from bombing *Borrelia* Lyme bacteria with antibiotics. Critics of alternative medicine bellow incessantly that people are swayed to use unproven methods that delay necessary medical care. But that doesn't fly here because most victims of tick-triggered illness have apparently already given conventional medicine more than its fair chance!

"I was having extreme fatigue, dizziness, joint pain, sinus, and digestive problems. I was missing a lot of work, and felt like it took all my energy just getting through the work day. I really enjoy running, and I used to be a professional figure skater. I'd be wiped out for days after a 2-mile run. [Prior to seeing Dr. Liebell], I was treated with anti-depressants, had all kinds of digestive tests done—for food allergies and gluten intolerance. I could tell within a few months that it [the BITE] was working, and continues to do so. It just takes time and perseverance. I can run up to 5 miles now, and not feel exhausted the next day! I'm planning on making a comeback in the skating world, but am too busy planning my wedding coming up in June! No more sinus problems... my joints don't hurt nearly as bad. I can tell my immune system is better; can't remember the last time I've been sick! Everything just seems easier. I'm sleeping better too. Antibiotics are evil! Although sometimes they are justified, most people take too many—then your immune system gets destroyed and you end up getting sick all the time...Homeopathy puts your immune system back in action"
                    - Jennifer W., Virginia Beach

Throughout this book I have carefully used the term tick-triggered illness rather than chronic Lyme disease. Although I am certain Lyme disease blood testing has its faults, I do agree that many suffering people do not have active chronic *Borrelia*

75

infection. They have illness *triggered* by it. The damage has been done, resulting in a complex cascade of imbalances and dysfunction of body systems, combined with susceptibility to countless other microbes and their subsequent effects.

Long-term antibiotic usage disturbs immune system function. Antibiotics can, of course be incredibly effective. However, when they succeed it is often because a healthy and strong enough immune system *finishes* the job, and prevents the infection's return. This is the key. If your immune system is impaired, it will be ill-equipped to handle the complex effects of tick-triggered and associated illness. The scientists and health governing bodies are clear in their stance that long-term antibiotics are both ineffective and dangerous. This is not the "Liebell hypothesis" of antibiotics. Safeguarding the public against antibiotic abuse is not part of some wild conspiracy to keep *Borrelia* alive.

The CDC state on their website (www.cdc.gov) that long-term antibiotic treatment for Lyme disease has been associated with serious complications, including death. This really hits home for me. Patty painfully stumbled her way into my office in 2010. Despite her rickety slow pace, and laundry list of symptoms, she radiated good cheer. Not bad for a lady in her sixties, who had been grimly diagnosed by other doctors with ALS (Lou Gehrig's disease) a life-threatening degenerative neurological condition. Patty was nevertheless optimistic when she consulted with me. I had not seen Patty for many years. She had come to me for chiropractic treatment periodically, and was hoping for some pain relief. She was a mere shadow of her former self. Upon telling me of her ALS diagnosis, I was immediately prompted to ask, *"Patty, have you ever been bitten by a tick?"* At first she thought it was a rhetorical question. Patty took frequent nature walks throughout her heavily-wooded golf course community, and had indeed pulled ticks off of herself on many an occasion. Most significantly, she had one that resulted in a huge bull's eye rash sprouting on her belly. This rash, which did not concern her family doctor one bit, came and went shortly before the onset of her ALS-associated symptoms. Yet none of the highly-credentialed physicians (including neurologists and rheumatologists) who evaluated Patty ever mentioned or considered Lyme disease!

Realistic hope at last, Patty thought. Finally, an unexpected and serendipitous opportunity to get better was on the horizon. The triggering cause of her cascading neurological symptoms was apparent. It made so much sense! Patty seemed to be quite excited and optimistic to begin her customized supportive holistic *natural* regimen. She brimmed with confidence that she now had a fighting chance, and *seemed* to be ready to roll. Sadly and mysteriously (and at the time unbeknownst to me), Patty had a change of heart. She was persuaded into taking aggressive antibiotic therapy instead. Despite two years of conventional physicians massively bungling both the diagnosis and treatment of her neurological disease, Patty put her trust in *them*. The supposedly Lyme savvy doctor put her on oral and intravenous antibiotics. She had one side effect after another…and died!

I was so saddened by her death. I didn't take her choice of treatment personally, but I will always wonder why didn't she trust me—the doctor who, in a matter of seconds, figured out what was *really* wrong with her? What a pity. I learned from a reliable source that the doctor, who assured her his antibiotic prescriptions were essential, was forced to retire by his state medical board. He chose to pack it in, rather than fight charges and sanctions for the overuse of antibiotics and painkillers. I can only speculate what unethical tactics he may have used to discourage Patty from pursuing *my* treatment. I am proud to have had the privilege to help many of the other patients who used to go to that particular doctor too. Maybe Patty would still be alive today. We will never know.

Your Body, Bacteria, and Your Immune System

Your body is composed of approximately 30 trillion human cells by DNA "head count." But you are not alone. Lurking throughout your body—sharing it as a shelter are an estimated 40 *trillion non-human cells!* That's right...you are outnumbered by microbes. Keep in mind that the average human cell is one hundred times larger than the average bacterial cell. A microscope is necessary to see bacteria. Viruses are even smaller than bacteria—they cannot be seen under a light microscope (an electron microscope is necessary). Viruses are 10 to 100 times *smaller* than bacteria. Other than size, what's the difference between bacteria and viruses? The biggest difference is that bacteria do not need a living surface to grow on. They live *in between* human cells. Viruses, on the other hand require a host cell—they live *inside* your cells. The word virus itself comes from Latin, meaning poison. All viruses are harmful (parasitic), but many bacteria are not only harmless, but essential and beneficial to your health.

You have as many as 1,000 species of microbes in your mouth alone. There are hundreds on your skin, and thousands in your intestines. Trying to kill them all is a <u>tragic mistake</u>. The notion that our best strategy for improving human health is to annihilate all species of bacteria is foolish on so many levels. Life on earth would not exist without bacteria.

Your health is dictated by how well your immune system handles the harmful bacteria, viruses, and other microorganisms.

Antibiotics are one of the pillars of modern medicine, and we are grateful for their existence. But you cannot continuously launch chemical weapons into your body, and expect a healthy result. You kill the good with the bad, and you don't just bounce back to normal. Recent scientific discoveries have been revealing the perils of antibiotic treatment. Thousands of people are dying each year from infections that antibiotics *used to* be able to cure! According to *Smithsonian* magazine (May 2013), early life exposure to antibiotics increases the likelihood of obesity, malnutrition, and central nervous system problems. They say mainstream medicine has been blindly tinkering with the microscopic world of our bodies for more than 70 years, since the dawn of the antibiotic era. Current science has revealed that the natural balance of healthful microorganisms struggles terribly to recover from repeated antibiotic assault, and that it has major health consequences. Lyme/antibiotic doctors suggest that taking probiotic supplements offset any damages. If only it were that simple!

Spirochaete Infection and Antibiotics

Syphilis is caused by a similar type bacterium of Lyme (spirochaete), *Treponema pallidum*. Patients with untreated or inadequately treated syphilis are notorious for suffering different stages. The bacteria can be present in your body for 10-30 years after infection! Symptoms can include problems with muscles, numbness, memory loss, mental illness, and problems with joints, etc. Scientists say spirochaete bacterial infections do NOT require long-term antibiotic therapy. It is a dangerous and unacceptable practice to prescribe antibiotics without evidence of active bacterial infection. This is why the term, "post treatment Lyme disease syndrome" has been suggested. There is no doubt that people suffer complex and progressive illness that is initiated by infection, long after active infection is gone.

"Unortho-Doxy"

What a luxury the manufacturers, marketers, stockholders, and prescribing physicians have—the public blindly accepts pharmaceutical drugs without question. Have you ever wondered what doxycycline is, and how it works, its risks, and who *shouldn't* be prescribed it? The authorities call it the cure for

Lyme disease. Innumerable patients do not concur. Nearly every one of them had taken it prior to seeing me. My *patients* are the critics of this drug. I have nothing to do with doxycycline on any level. I don't prescribe it, nor do I ever *un*-prescribe it.

"Doxy?" That's the jargon of the Lyme community. I cringe when I hear a powerful and potentially hazardous pharmaceutical drug referred to in such a casual and practically *affectionate* manner. A nickname? Really? There is nothing cute and cuddly about doxycycline. It is not a Teddy bear! The Internet has various threads about *suicide* related to "doxy" use. More than 10,000 people have reported side effects, and more than 100 have died. Pregnant women and children under 8-years-old are not supposed to take it (it can impair their bone growth and cause brain swelling), but it is still sometimes prescribed to them! Doxycycline has been implicated with development of inflammatory bowel disease such as Crohn's disease, among other risky considerations.

I read the medical journals. Published side effects of doxycycline include life-threatening allergic reactions, blood problems, liver damage, erosion of the esophagus, nausea, vomiting, diarrhea, increased sensitivity of the skin to sunlight, yeast infection, and *dozens* of others. Has your doctor told you that doxycycline can interfere with your calcium and iron levels? What about its effect on the function of birth control pills (it can make them not work)?

I spend a lot of time educating people in the principles of homeopathic and bio-energetic medicine—sadly having to *defend* internationally-accepted, holistic health care methods, which have NO side effects or drug interactions. What I would appreciate is that antibiotic treatment—specifically doxycycline doesn't get a free ride.

Crossing the Blood-Brain-Barrier

Those of us, who have scoured the Internet and every other resources for help with Lyme disease are familiar with the term, "blood-brain-barrier." Throughout our bodies, we have capillaries (our smallest blood vessels), which have a lining of specialized cells (endothelial). These endothelial cells are tightly fitted together to form a filter. This is a feature of our anatomy and physiology that acts as a blocking wall or filter to prevent harmful substances from getting into the brain and spinal cord. It protects the brain by preventing large molecules from passing through to it. However, the blood-brain-barrier can be weakened by various illnesses, radiation, infection, and trauma.

The blood-brain-barrier makes it tough for medications to reach the brain. This is mostly a good thing because we don't want harmful chemicals in our brains! Antibiotic molecules are typically too large to cross the blood-brain-barrier. If they do get through, it is thought that they cannot penetrate in large enough quantity to have the desired effect. This makes infections of the brain difficult to treat. Although weakening of the blood-brain-barrier may make it possible for some antibiotics to break through, it is highly questionable whether or not it is safe for them to be there! Perhaps you've been told that herbal remedies such as teasel, cat's claw, or Samento, were good for Lyme. While some people have found them symptomatically helpful, it is likely most of their molecules cannot cross the blood-brain-barrier either.

If you have been on antibiotics for years, in an effort to recover from Lyme, perhaps you will want to consider this information wisely. If Lyme *Borrelia* bacteria, as well as *Bartonella, Ehrlicia, Babesia,* and *Toxoplasma* are living in your brain, can antibiotics likely kill them? This question does not even take into account the antibiotic resistant nature of many bacteria species.

Biofilm Barricade Busting

Biofilm is another one of the many debated topics in Lyme treatment. **Biofilm** is a protective slimy coated matrix of bacteria. It makes the microbes resistant to antibiotics, as well as herbal medicine. The Lyme community obsesses over biofilm. I do not. It is not a concern when implementing our holistic homeopathic approach. Human bodies have been successfully dealing with biofilm for as long as we have walked the planet. Most bacterial infections involve biofilms, which provide resistance to antibiotics. The *National Institutes of Health* and the CDC report that more than 80 percent of ALL bacterial infections include a biofilm phase during the course of the disease (grants.nih.gov)

The bio-energetic medicine approach (which you will learn about later on) is not in any way limited or challenged by biofilm. Quite frankly, discussions of such do not enter in the equation for my patients as a factor in analysis, diagnosis, treatment, or recovery. When my patients feel their memory restored, their joint and muscle pains disappear, and their energy return, they no longer give a second thought about biofilm.

Medications Meddling with Metals

You may already be aware that antibiotics kill the normal beneficial bacteria in your gut. What you might not know is that in healthy people, these bacteria serve the vital function of carting away poisonous metals such as aluminum, lead, mercury, copper, and cadmium. This is nothing to sneeze at. As you learned earlier, just one of these metals can cause nearly every symptom you've associated with Lyme disease! Therefore, this is of grave concern if you have been taking doxycycline for any extended period of time (or cycling different antibiotics). This is another reason why your focus must shift away from bombing bacteria over to supporting your <u>immune system</u>.

It is true. ALL steroids suppress the immune system. Acetaminophen is a popular drug, consumed like candy that can interfere with liver function. Reduced liver function decreases removal of toxins caused by infection. Although drugs for heartburn (gastro-esophageal reflux) are designed to block stomach acid secretion, they also inhibit the immune system, which can increase risk of infection, such as pneumonia! Antidepressant drugs are prescribed and taken with reckless abandon in America. How often do doctors tell their patients that these drugs may be one of the many triggers for autoimmune disease? What about opioid drugs like codeine, oxycodone, fentanyl, or morphine? Can these also suppress your immune system? You bet they can!

The "Peeling Layers of an Onion" Paradigm Predicament

Peeling layers of the onion? The concept is that in a highly-structured and order-dependent fashion, one must separately and sequentially address each microorganism, toxin, or organ problem. I have encountered countless patients who were told by other doctors that they must first aggressively detoxify the liver, kidneys, colon, gall bladder, and so forth prior to going after microbes. Others insist heavy metal detoxification must be done first. Still others insist upon "parasite cleanses," or addressing *Borrelia* with doxycycline before trying to annihilate *Bartonella* or *Mycoplasma* with a different drug or herb. Then it's on trying to kill the fungi or the worms or some other species, family, or kingdom of life.

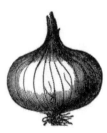

83

Human beings are not onions in need of peeling! To some degree, I once too subscribed to this philosophy. However, through my experience with lots of patients, I discovered it simply was not accurate, nor was it necessary. While it is accurate to say recovery, rehabilitation, or repair can sometimes naturally take place within the body in stages—one must not arrogantly assume it can be *intellectually* determined what to try to kill in the body, and in what order. Our bodies do not operate physiologically one function at a time. All cells, tissues, and organs work together constantly as one cohesive and synchronized unit. In health, the immune system is constantly attempting to manage all microbes and other irritants. It must be capable of effectively functioning as a whole.

The general philosophy of many Lyme-centered treatment approaches is academic in nature. With the *Bio-Energetic Individual Treatment Equation*, we hold the internal inborn wisdom of the human body in much higher regard. We must strive to improve overall function all at once—without shocking or antagonizing the body. With the BITE, we do not peel away layers of the onion. Creating a customized, whole-body, wellness-based protocol (discussed in later chapters) is an all-at-once health approach. We humans are not machines, nor are we onions.

Staying Clear from the Controversy... and Getting People Healthy

In closing out this chapter, please consider that this book is *not* for people who have succeeded with antibiotic therapy. I am sincerely happy for those lucky ones for whom treatment was so simple and easy. I neither condemn nor condone those who chose to take that approach. I have never, and will never suggest to any patient, prospective patient, or reader that conventional medical care should be avoided. By no means am I suggesting that anybody with a medically-confirmed active infection should not see a doctor, who may prescribe antibiotics.

My family and I make choices, and I provide advice for my patients based upon science, safety, and RESULTS. So should you. There is no need to feel torn between conventional and holistic medical approaches because they should coexist and complement each other. Beware of Lyme-ignorant doctors and those who view chronic pain and illness as a one-size-fits-all problem to diagnose and treat with antibiotics, painkillers, antidepressants, and anti-inflammatory drugs.

The apparent Lyme disease crisis is not a matter of insurance coverage and support for long-term antibiotic usage. It is the failure to focus on the prevention of disease and promotion of wellness, in favor of treating the effects of disease. Doctors seem to rely on only one familiar tool, as stated in the Law of the Instrument by psychologist, Abraham Maslow: *"I suppose it is tempting, if the only tool you have is a hammer, to treat everything as if it were a nail."*

(Source: *Abraham H. Maslow (1966), The Psychology of Science, p.15*)

Drugs are the most common "hammer" utilized in American health care. There's a drug for every symptom and condition. Antibiotics are supposed to hammer away Lyme disease. I cannot know with complete certainty the extent to which they do or not. What I do know is that throughout my ongoing study of the subject of Lyme disease, I consistently find scientists emphatically urging doctors to only prescribe antibiotics for patients who have serious active bacterial infections. The role of antibiotics is suggested as a means of tipping the balance in favor of patients' own immune system defenses.

Misuse and abuse of one of the most important tools in the history of medicine has caused this crisis. Yet the battle cry of the chronic Lyme community is to let doctors prescribe long-term antibiotics to potentially millions of Americans. This would contribute further to a raging predicament. And most importantly, it is completely unnecessary!

Antibiotics are certainly magnificent medicines, which can save lives. Nevertheless, they must not be used as rampantly and casually as over-the-counter painkillers. Yet, they continue to be utilized as such. It has become common knowledge that taking antibiotics (particularly long-term) is harmful to the body. Martin J. Blaser, M.D., the director of the *Human Microbiome Program* at *New York University* has produced a mountain of overwhelming scientific evidence that overuse of antibiotics is dangerous—far beyond the threat of antibiotic-resistant infections. Dr. Blaser makes a provocative and rational case in his book, *Missing Microbes: How the Overuse of Antibiotics Is Fueling Our Modern Plagues*. He explains the science behind his declaration that excessive antibiotics usage is one of the major causes of today's expanded levels of chronic illnesses. This includes food allergies, asthma, gastrointestinal disorders, diabetes, and even some forms of cancer. In his book, Dr. Blaser explains why doctors must use extreme caution with antibiotics, and that patients should consider alternative methods.

During our correspondence, Dr. Blaser and I discussed how antibiotics are extremely important when *appropriately* used. I concurred that giving patients long and potentially dangerous courses of antibiotics was a bad practice for those without real evidence of infection. Dr. Blaser was glad I could help people with my approach.

86

Scientists are aware that there are one hundred or more unknown bacterial species that live inside us. The consequences of indiscriminately killing them are not yet known. It is *absolutely* known that bacteria contribute to essential functions of the human body. The report, *Antibiotic resistance threats in the United States, 2013* provides us for the first time with a glimpse at the serious burden and threats posed by the most significant antibiotic-resistant germs. In this report, the CDC estimate that in the United States, more than two million people become ill from antibiotic-resistant infection, with at least 23,000 dying as a result. Here's an Internet link to the actual report, should you be interested in reading it:

http://www.cdc.gov/drugresistance/threat-report-2013/pdf/ar-threats-2013-508.pdf

In the history of the world, especially pre-dating science, explanations of natural phenomena have always changed over time. The very nature of science is to constantly strive for better explanations and understanding of what we observe and experience in life. Human history proves constantly that whoever is in currently in power tends to hold the definitive explanation. The world was once most certainly flat—according to some of the finest minds of the day.

I was born in 1966. During my lifetime I have observed the ever-changing gospel of weight loss. At one time calories were the rage. Then the focus went to the number of grams of fat, and later the wrong kind of fat. The low-carb craze eventually took over, refined later by the glycemic index. Eggs were good, eggs were bad, and now they're good again. Diets, fads, gadgets, and celebrity trainers come and go. Antibiotics were once predicted to be the cure for all disease, and now scientists are discovering they may have become a *cause!* Truths in medicine are relative to time. The one constant has been, and always will be that the body heals itself when free of interference. Ancient cultures knew this before the study of anatomy and physiology was conceived at a scientific level. Our bodies are capable at overcoming infection. Not all infection, all the time—but most of the time. For many decades, antibiotics have been boasted as the cure for disease. Some time, perhaps not in the too distant future we will look back at the era of antibiotics and exclaim, *"What were we thinking?"*

According to a 2018 report from the Infectious Diseases Society of America (2018), outpatient antibiotic overprescribing is rampant. Nearly half of the antibiotic prescriptions are written without infection diagnosis! This study of more than half a million prescriptions from 514 clinics revealed clinicians prescribed antibiotics without an infection-related diagnosis nearly half of the time. One in five prescriptions were provided without an in-person visit. These antibiotic prescriptions were found to be made for either a bad reason, or no reason at all!

Jeffrey A. Linder, MD, MPH, Chief, Division of General Internal Medicine and Geriatrics, Northwestern University Feinberg School of Medicine, Chicago

Chapter 10

The Detoxification Abomination

Why You Must Not Forcefully "Detox"

Detoxification and drainage are critical to a wellness-based approach to recovery from chronic tick-triggered illness. However, it must not be forceful. In my opinion, many popular detoxification methods are disastrous, painful, unhealthy, and ill-advised. Gently supporting your body to naturally and gradually eliminate toxins *itself*—is a critical part of recovery with the BITE. More than ever before in human history, we are exposed to chemical toxins. Our bodies are relentlessly bombarded by toxic substances from countless sources. They are in our food and water supply, and the air we breathe. Prescription and over-the-counter medications have many toxic ingredients. Building materials, household cleaning products, and numerous other sources one might never consider are laden with toxins. For example, a plastic beverage container may be composed of chemicals which end up in its liquid contents. A toxic effect can come from electromagnetic radiation. We may not like to learn that cell phones, computers, and high voltage electric power lines can emit toxic levels of radiation, but it is a fact. Toxins from infectious microorganisms add to the sinister mix.

The human body naturally eliminates toxins that result from normal metabolism. It has sophisticated detoxification and drainage systems. However, everybody has a breaking point where a toxic overload is no longer effectively handled by the organs responsible. The consequences differ tremendously from person to person. Symptoms can range from fatigue to serious illness. The organs of detoxification and drainage include the lymphatic vessels and lymph nodes, liver, kidneys, bowels, skin, and the lungs. Many of your symptoms may be at least in part, caused by toxic overload.

Conventional Western medicine is rather uncomfortable with this. A visit to a conventional American medical doctor rarely involves a conversation regarding toxins. The focus is on symptoms, diagnosis (a name for your symptoms), and typically prescriptions for medication to alleviate your symptoms. Do you think a regimen of long-term antibiotics addresses mobilization and elimination of toxic substances in your body? The drugs themselves are additional toxins for your body to deal with.

In my practice, I have access to the same detoxification products as any other doctor. My typical patient has already failed to improve after implementing a wide variety of flushes, cleanses, and detoxification regimens. Imagine having a plumber clean out the pipes of your home's sewage system, but neglect to *repair* or replace anything that is broken, which caused the crud accumulation. The clogs and backups will return in no time. Forcing toxins out of the body may seem like a good idea, however detoxification and drainage is a process which should be naturally taking place all the time!

The secret to my patients' success has been restoring their natural detoxification systems. We do not aggressively try to rapidly clean them out. I do not advocate herbal cleanses and complicated nutritional approaches. Like antibiotics, aggressive colon cleanses and "detox" flushes may interfere with the normal balance of gut flora. We need gut bacteria for digestion of food, synthesis of vitamins, and removal of toxins. I have found these approaches to be too harsh, more expensive, risky, and quite frankly, far less effective than the right combination of bio-energetic homeopathic supports for each individual (discussed in later chapters). The goal is having the body eliminate toxins itself from the cells outward, in a natural manner. Natural does not mean forcing them out rapidly by introducing a physical or chemical force. It means normal physiology. This is readily observed. For those who have been exposed to complex and aggressive detoxification regimens, this might sound unrealistic and too simplistic. It is quite the opposite. The human body's systems of detoxification are magnificently complex and breathtakingly capable—with the right support. With merely a "gentle push," rather than an aggressive plunging, detoxification can be achieved by the body itself. Unfortunately, some people find this simple concept hard to believe. That is their prerogative.

MTHFR?

The study of genetics is fascinating, important, and can lead to life-saving developments. There are, however circumstances where science does not necessary facilitate progress. Many people are stifled by the assumption that they cannot detoxify because of a recently discovered genetic mutation associated with **methyl-tetrahydrofolate reductase** (MTHFR). This is an enzyme involved in cellular detoxification. The research suggests that those with certain variations of the MTHFR mutation will have a harder time eliminating toxins from their cells. My response to this is that knowledge of this genetic factor must not hold us back from the pursuit of wellness. Should those who get tested positive for this just give up? This is another battlefield on which I do not recommend fighting. What good will it do? My suspicion is that countless humans have this mutation, who are living healthfully. I have not seen its presence impede patient progress under my care, nor has it been necessary to make any special changes in anybody's treatment protocol at the present time.

91

"It began with a burning pain and stiffness in my neck, followed by muscle aches, heart palpitations, trembling, leg spasms, blurred vision, and panic attacks. Additionally, burning sensation and ringing in my ears... I was unable to concentrate at work, and had to reduce my hours... I felt like I was losing control of my life and the ability to do simple things. I felt like a failure. Since Dr. Liebell's treatment, I have been able to get back to all my activities, work full days, and enjoy the things my illness prevented me from doing. I can now do everything I was able to before my illness. It was an easy form of pain and drug free testing that required very little on my part. Do NOT give up hope, be patient, and let the treatment program do its job."

- Rory G., Seattle, WA

Chapter 11

Sleep Cycle Sadness & Melatonin Madness

Lack of proper sleep can contribute to a variety of medical problems. It can affect virtually any aspect of your health. Most victims of tick-triggered illness have a serious sleep debt. This means an accumulated lack of sleep over many months or years. Living things have 24-hour internal clocks known as **circadian rhythms.** Your internal clock enables you to adapt to your environment. It is a driving force for all the cells of your body. Any interference to the circadian rhythm has a cumulative effect on your health. Getting one or two good night's sleep cannot even the debt. Your body repairs and regenerates during sleep. It is therefore critical to take it seriously. Your ability to fight off illness depends not just on the quantity of your sleep, but more importantly the *quality*. I have observed that many people peculiarly take *pride* in being sleep deprived! This is a disturbing trend—bragging about working (and playing) too hard and too long. This is actually a conscious decision to decrease one's health.

We are diurnal beings. This means it is natural for us to sleep when it gets dark and wake up when it gets light. This is of course, no brilliant observation, yet it is largely not followed. Many people suffer circadian rhythm disturbances, resulting in physiological confusion in the body. It is notable that sleep disorders and deprivation can result in hormonal imbalances linked to obesity. Although there is considerable disagreement among researchers on the question of how much sleep we need, there is no disputing that people need quality, quantity, and consistency.

Following the Herd

When it comes to health, doing what everybody else is doing is the road to ruin. Prescription and over-the-counter sleep medicine is Western medicine's answer to sleep difficulties. Using drugs as a primary approach to sleep dysfunction has no scientific basis. In my opinion, it is a frightening and barbaric practice. Applying a brute force attack to induce drowsiness does not restore a normal healthy sleep cycle. Some of the serious potential side effects from some of the most popular prescription sleep drugs include: amnesia, hallucinations and delusions, coordination difficulty, increased appetite, decreased sex drive, and impaired judgment. There have been reports of people not remembering activities such as driving a car, eating, talking on the phone, having sex, and sleep walking.

Correcting the causes of sleep troubles takes much more than merely prescribing a drug. It takes serious detective work. Sleep disturbances are often an effect of other underlying medical conditions. There are many possible reasons for poor sleep. One major problem is low production of the essential hormone, melatonin. Melatonin is produced by the pineal gland, which is located in the brain.

The Pineal Gland & Your Health

The pineal gland is a pea-sized brain structure that has only recently been known to have great importance to many bodily functions. It gets its name from its pine cone shape (Latin *pinea*). This "master gland" responds to different levels of light, and thus is instrumental in your biological clock. It regulates the sleep cycles, as well

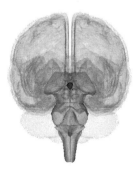

as sexual development. The pineal gland transforms the neurotransmitter, serotonin (the "happiness" chemical) into the hormone, melatonin. Frightfully ironic it is that pineal gland function can be disrupted by antidepressant drugs! Knowledge of such a fact makes it challenging not to feel bitter towards our medical system.

Running on Empty

Your melatonin production takes place only when it is dark. When light strikes the retina of your eye, nerve impulses to the pineal gland <u>shut down</u> melatonin production. It appears that pineal gland and melatonin are not only involved in sleep, but other aspects of our health, including fertility and aging. People diagnosed with Seasonal Affective Disorder (SAD) should know about the pineal gland. Researchers hypothesize that it has greater physiological importance than ever considered. Melatonin production tends to decrease with age.

Melatonin pills are sold as a natural supplement to treat insomnia, depression, and jet lag. This is a deceptive practice. Normal regulation and production of melatonin is unlikely to be restored by giving the body melatonin. The pineal gland must perform its functions by producing and regulating hormones itself. Taking melatonin hormone supplements may actually suppress normal pineal function. It is hardly a healthy long-term solution, and thus I do not advocate it. I would never give my patients melatonin, even though countless professionals applaud this "natural" approach to sleep. Melatonin supplements may be derived from nature—but they are <u>not</u> natural.

Make it Yourself!

To achieve better sleep, your pineal gland must naturally regulate melatonin levels. This results in truly restorative sleep that regenerates both mind and body. You can help increase

95

your body's *production* of melatonin by eating raw whole foods such as pineapples, bananas, cherries, tomatoes, and oranges. Whole raw walnuts are another melatonin-supportive food. Vitamin B6-rich foods are helpful for your body to generate its own melatonin. Fish such as salmon and tuna are excellent sources of B6. Dark green leafy vegetables like spinach and kale are rich in calcium, which is important in your body's manufacturing of melatonin. These are foods that most folks should be eating anyway!

In my practice, patients receive auricular therapy (ear acupuncture treatment) and bio-energetic homeopathic supplementation to support pineal (and other glandular) function. Bedtime rituals must be addressed with each individual patient. It is critical to treat the person instead of the "sleep disorder." Many people simply don't have enough energy to support and sustain their own sleep cycles. Add to this, anxiety, stress, and worries, which can be part of having a hyperactive mind and body. This is complicated further by regular use of substances like caffeine and alcohol. Rarely considered by doctors, but tremendously important is undetected toxicity and infection. Microorganisms can affect the pineal gland, as can various toxic chemicals. The sodium fluoride added to public water supplies may cause calcification of the pineal gland. Fluoride is an entire topic of great controversy and concern, for which I encourage investigation.

Prescription sleep medications fly off the shelves, while the cause of the problem isn't even remotely considered (let alone treated). Addressing the causes of sleep problems is an essential part of the *Bio-energetic Individual Treatment Equation.*© We must address regulation of hormones and neurotransmitters. We must address underlying causes of stress and illness, and take our time to find realistic solutions (and realistic time frameworks to achieve them).

Sleep Cycle Support
Through the Ear Gateway

Using the fascinating and sophisticated techniques of Auricular Bio-energetic Testing (ABT), we commonly find energetic blockages to the pineal gland. These are quickly and safely corrected by means of 3-phase auricular therapy, using neuro-electric ear stimulation and/or needle acupuncture. Incidentally, the pineal gland cannot be *directly* affected by meridian-based traditional Chinese acupuncture. Acupuncture performed on pinpoint areas detected on the ear, which directly correspond by reflex with the pineal gland and other sleep-related brain structures can jumpstart the restoration of normal circadian rhythm. ABT and auricular therapy are explained in detail in later chapters.

It is critical to address correction of sleep cycles, but not to attempt to chemically induce drowsiness with medicine. Causing drowsiness is the single-minded pharmacological approach. Even though I passionately disagree with the philosophy, I do not tell patients to discontinue usage of prescription sleep aids without discussing it with the prescribing physician. The goal is to safely and gradually reduce the need for sleep medication over time as cycles are normalized. The homeopathic bio-energetic supplements I provide do not deliver doses of pharmaceutical medicine, but rather energetic essences of various substances, designed to support normal sleep cycle regulation. Details of the ear acupuncture and this method will be discussed in later chapters.

If you suffer chronic pain, sleep difficulties may play a large role in preventing recovery. I am proud to safely and sensibly address this aspect of my patients' health in a unique manner. It's not as simple as inserting an acupuncture needle in a "sleep point." Every patient is evaluated for energetic blockages of the pineal gland and several other brain structures. Comprehensive case history and consideration of sleep cycles and rituals is an essential component of whole-body, wellness-based treatment.

Sleeping can be a Nightmare

For many patients, the challenge of sleep lies in suffering from an overactive mind at bedtime. Many people feel exhausted both physically and mentally, but when it comes down to going to bed—they simply cannot turn off their own brain. Their own thoughts keep them awake, ruminating over the events of the day, the day before, and what is going on tomorrow. Bedtime is sleepy time; it is not problem solving time. But many suffer the inability to shut down their own thoughts. Waking up many times during the night can start the whole maddening and frustrating process over again and again.

Have you ever fallen asleep on the couch or bed watching television? You probably were not *trying* to fall asleep, so there was no pressure or conscious effort to do so. You just did. But then, you got up and tucked yourself into bed to *intentionally* go to sleep—but it was a disaster. Your mind was set on the goal of falling asleep. Maybe this happens to you on a regular basis. Here's a suggestion:

Have Someone Read
You a Bedtime Story

Reading children bedtime stories is a time-tested method that has worked beautifully for generations. It can work equally as well for adults too. The secret is listening to audiobooks. Bedtime story time is right at your fingertips, and if you are willing... it is FREE! I have seen this to be effective for over 25 years. You can get thousands of titles of recorded books on CD from most local public library systems. You can also purchase them from bookstores and online stores very easily. My public library system here in Virginia Beach even has instant download audiobooks that can be legally imported to an mp3 player, IPod, or whatever device you have. Perhaps your regional library system has the same type service. When you listen to a recorded book, it provides a distraction from your own thoughts. It can help you fall asleep because when you are listing to a story, you are not *trying* to sleep. Many people listen to books that they do not have time to read. Other alternatives include podcasts, which are available by the thousands on the Web. It is important that the listening material does not include music, commercials, or any fluctuating volume.

Core Biting Back Principle: Restoring healthy sleep cycles requires normal function of the pineal gland. This cannot be accomplished by taking melatonin supplements. Ear acupuncture (auricular therapy) and bio-energetic supplementation are the means by which we support the body to restore pineal gland function itself.

Chapter 12

Treatment with Rife? Not on Your Life!

The Rife machine is a device familiar to many who have searched for Lyme solutions. It was invented around 1930 by Royal Raymond Rife. He suggested that all cancer was caused by bacteria. Although one bacterial species, *Helicobacter pylori* has indeed been linked to stomach cancer, science has revealed viruses (such as Epstein Barr) and fungi to be more significant culprits. Rife machines are proposed to generate radio frequencies that kill bacteria by vibrating them until they explode. Blasting the bacteria with killing frequencies instead of using antibiotic chemical warfare might seem like an interesting idea, but it has flaws which exclude from being part of the *Bio-energetic Individualized Treatment Equation*.

Herxheimer Hoax?

Rife machine users believe bacteria are being killed because they seem to experience Jarisch-Herxheimer reactions. Often referred to as "herxing," Herxheimer reactions are a side effect of antibiotic treatment. Dead or injured bacteria suddenly release their internal toxins directly into the blood stream at a pace that is overwhelming to the body. The patient sufferers a highly-exaggerated inflammatory response that can feel like an intense worsening of the existing condition. Herxheimer reactions were originally observed in antibiotic treatment of syphilis in the late 1890s. Some Lyme/antibiotic-focused doctors suggest the Herxheimer reactions constitute proof of chronic bacterial infection when laboratory diagnosis suggests otherwise.

Most sufferers of tick-triggered illness have seriously impaired systems of detoxification and drainage. Even if Rife machines do indeed kill bacteria, an ailing body is ill-equipped to cope with a rapid onslaught of die-off toxins. *Any* treatment that causes rapid die-off can further stress an already overwhelmed system. Like antibiotics, I do not think Rife frequency treatment *strengthens* the body, nor does it support immune system regulation. If the body's natural systems are not better functioning; the patient is not better. Furthermore, Rife machines are <u>not</u> FDA-cleared medical devices either. I will not use any treatment that could potentially harm anybody. Years ago, I observed that those patients who used the Rife machine (on their own accord), in conjunction with my treatment did not achieve satisfactory results. The Rife machine undermined their success! While blowing up bacteria with killing frequencies may sound like a good idea as an alternative to antibiotics, I sternly warn against it. I am aware that testimonials of people who have succeeded with Rife treatment exist, and I think it is worth further scientific exploration for other uses. Nevertheless, it is off-limits during my care.

I never have, nor will I ever interfere with a patient's prescription medical treatment. Patients who seek my wellness care for tick-triggered illness, typically have tried and failed with antibiotic therapy. Some begin my treatment while still on antibiotics, and by their own decision wean themselves off them. I let them know that it's safe and okay to do both types of treatment, although it will take much longer to get better. I do not ever tell anybody to stop antibiotics. However, I do insist that anybody seeking my care discontinues usage of the Rife machine. I am not trying to criticize patients and doctors or their treatment choices. My duty is to educate. My mission is to restore health to those in need. I could easily get Rife machines for my patients and sell them for a tidy profit. I do not, and I will not. Not for the Rife of me!

Taking your Rife in Your Hands?
The top 7 reasons to NOT Use Rife machines

1. Rife machines use powerful KILLING frequencies—not HEALING frequencies, therefore their usage does not promote wellness

2. Rife treatment does NOT (to my knowledge) enhance immune system function—it is just another proposed "weapon of mass destruction" intended to directly annihilate microbes. TRUE health and progressive strengthening of the body must come as a result of your immune system attacking germs.

3. Rife treatment seems to cause rapid die-off release of toxins, which results in the significant side effects associated with Herxheimer reactions caused by antibiotics.

4. Like antibiotic therapy, Rife treatment does not account for detoxification or drainage of such toxins.

5. Rife machines are also a large and unnecessary expense.

6. Rife machines are not FDA approved devices for medical use. I will not potentially endanger my patients' health, nor will I use a device that is not legal for my usage.

7. I repeatedly see patients for whom Rife treatment has failed. I have found that success is absolutely hindered by these machines! I'm not saying Rife machines don't ever work... they simply do not improve MY patients' results... they make them worse, in my experience.

Chapter 13

The Glutathione Gluttony Glorification

There are tens of thousands of medical articles available in support of the importance of **glutathione**. Your body produces this detoxifying antioxidant molecule that is composed of three amino acids: cysteine, glycine and glutamine. Amino acids are the building blocks of protein. Without boring you with a chemistry lesson, you should know that the term, **antioxidant**, refers to chemicals that prevent the formation of cell damaging substances called **free radicals**. Many harmful substances get stuck to glutathione molecules, which is why it is important for detoxification. And yes, chronically ill people have been observed to exhibit low levels of glutathione.

Do you *really* need to obsess over this antioxidant to get better? My observation has been that the Lyme disease community has been trained to do so. Glutathione supplementation is a major focus of antibiotic-centered chronic Lyme protocols. Why? Perhaps it is because scientific studies have shown that a side effect of antibiotic therapy may be reduced glutathione levels!

I do not suggest that glutathione supplements are harmful, but rather that they are an unnecessary expense. My natural and holistic wellness treatments do not involve antibiotics, thus no such supplementation is necessary to try to counter side effects. Taking whole glutathione supplements is questionably effective for increasing your body's levels. The vast majority of my patients have come to me after lengthy Lyme protocols that included substantial glutathione supplementation, at significant cost—with no improvement. Many practitioners suggest consuming truckloads of nutrient pills constitutes natural health

103

care. I dispute this with a passion. Natural does not simply mean that one is not using drugs. Why flush money down the drain with expensive supplements when you can ensure greater nutrition and nutrient absorption through foods? Spend your hard-earned money on the highest quality of nutritious whole foods you can afford. You have to eat—so why not get your nutrition the truly natural way?

Glutathione supplementation is *not* a concern within the *Bio-energetic Individual Treatment Equation*©. It is preferable for your body to naturally manufacture this antioxidant itself. I recommend eating whole foods providing the *building blocks* of glutathione. Excellent sources include kale, broccoli, watercress, asparagus, collard greens, and cauliflower. Foods rich in vitamin C support glutathione production too. This includes the green food (which actually provide it better than the long-coveted citrus fruits). Peppers are one of the best vitamin C sources you can eat. However, one must avoid high doses of vitamin C. According to cancer specialist, Yoshiaki Omura, MD, overconsumption of vitamin C cancels the cancer-fighting benefits of vitamin D3! A high-quality whey protein powder can be incorporated into outstanding whole food breakfast shakes. The Liebell family has been doing so for years. Glutathione levels can also be boosted by exercise, but please do not do so at the expense of harming your progress! Most people I treat are in no condition to begin exercise programs yet.

Never Too Old to Get Well

"I suffered dizziness, confusion, and fatigue. I avoided family and friends, and limited my activity. I couldn't do line dancing or go to social events. I went to medical doctors, psychiatrists, psychologists, sleep therapists, and Lyme literate medical doctors with no success. Since Dr. Liebell's treatment, my social life has improved. I was able to make a trip to Florida to attend my granddaughter's graduation! I've got more energy and improved sleep. Dr. Liebell is so caring, encouraging and confident.

- Shirley M., Virginia Beach

Chapter 14:

Taking the Rut Out of Leaky Gut

Leaky gut is popular jargon among nutritionists and more enlightened doctors. It refers to expansion of openings in the intestinal lining, which results in partially digested food particles and other substances leaking inappropriately into the bloodstream. The true medical term is **intestinal hyper-permeability**. Picture a strainer that is supposed to have small fine openings that have spread out larger, enabling larger particles to get through. The key functions of the small intestines are breakdown and absorption of nutrients from food that arrive from the stomach. With a leaky gut, incompletely digested molecules of foods and waste products that would not normally pass through the intestinal "strainer" leak into the bloodstream. Your body reacts to these substances as if they were harmful foreign invaders. This is thought to create excessive stress on the liver to deal with ongoing wastes that tightly-pored intestines would prevent. Inflammation in various body tissues can be the dreadful result. It has been hypothesized that autoimmune diseases may be triggered by this.

It seems obvious that many new food allergies could crop up as a result of increased intestinal permeability. An otherwise healthful food can become an irritant because some of its undigested particles can inappropriately enter the bloodstream. It is not the food itself that is the cause of the allergy, but rather the body's impaired function and the subsequent response that is the problem. One may be deprived of some of the nutrients the food would normally provide if completely digested.

Demystifying Leaky Gut Syndrome

One of the greatest obstacles towards recovery can be information overload. Sometimes knowledge, or over-thinking a problem creates a disadvantage. Cries of leaky gut, as well as gluten intolerance have in my opinion, been vastly overstated. Bookstores and the Internet are loaded with nutritional approaches to leaky gut. Not this book! The road to health is paved by supporting your body to naturally deal with the parasites that cause the leaky gut in the first place!

This is a topic for which there is no consistent agreement throughout the medical community. There are those who deny its existence, as well as varying opinions of its causes and how to address it. Leaky gut has been associated with more obvious problems such as symptoms of the gastrointestinal system, but also arthritis, skin problems, allergies, and others. It is my suspicion that doctors do not like the concept of leaky gut because it does not conform to the named condition-based concept of conventional medicine. Like Lyme disease, leaky gut may be something that can cause (not mimic) all kinds of popular named conditions for which FDA-approved drug intervention is accepted as standard treatment. There is no drug for leaky gut syndrome. It is technically not a real diagnosis.

The consequences of leaky gut can be different for each person, with different body tissues being affected. Those who develop food sensitivities or allergies may be actually developing antibodies to nearly everything being eaten. The immune system may respond to the food particles leaking through as they were *parasites*! Some people develop skin rashes, which are the result of the body eliminating toxins. Others suffer headaches, fatigue, memory troubles, anxiety, and nearly every symptom a human can suffer. Doctors can undoubtedly diagnose various *other* conditions for which a popular drug can indefinitely be prescribed for symptomatic management!

Questioning the Nutritional Supplement Approach

I rarely encounter a patient who has <u>not</u> previously tried extensive nutritional supplementation, as well as probiotics in an attempt to remedy both the leaky gut problems, as well as other effects of tick-triggered illness. My patients have learned through experience that gobbling down massive quantities of supplements every day does not solve the problem. Mega-doses of vitamins, minerals, amino acids, and enzymes do not address the causes of the expanded porous opening of the intestines that are obstructing normal nutrient absorption. Nor do they mobilize the immune system to attack the sources of the intestinal leakage. I mean no harm or criticism of other professionals, nor do I represent my opinions and methods as the end-all, cure-all. My commentary is based upon consistent personal and patient experiences. I do not accept that people are suddenly allergic to foods simply because of preservatives, genetic modification, and other chemical contributors. Nor is stress likely a direct cause. These are indeed bad things, but I do not view them as critical as others do. I have my reasons, which I shall share with you.

The Causes of Leaky Gut Doctors are Reluctant to Mention

Expansion of the openings in the intestine can be triggered by many things, particularly infection. **All Lyme disease-obsessed doctors and patients must be aware that *antibiotics* cause inflammation and damage to the lining of your intestines, which allow toxic bowel waste products to enter your bloodstream!** Historically, the only other way this would happen would be through trauma, particularly a stab wound from a spear or sword! Both antibiotics and non-steroidal anti-inflammatory drugs (Aleive, Advil, Motrin, etc.)

107

cause the spaces of the intestines to widen, which results in leaky gut syndrome. When substances that shouldn't leak into your bloodstream are absorbed—it leads to symptoms often diagnosed as arthritis or fibromyalgia.

Do Parasites Cause the Leaky Gut...?
Or Does the Leaky Gut Cause Parasitic Infection?

It is like the old question, *"What came first...the chicken or the egg?"* FYI: the scientific answer is indeed the *egg*—but that is a subject for another book! Here we are wondering if the parasites cause the leaky gut, or if it is the other way around. While it likely depends upon the individual, we do know that parasites damage the lining of the intestines, which causes leaky gut. No matter which comes first, it is critical to overcome chronic infection in order to improve leaky gut.

How Do We Get Parasites?

Parasites are everywhere, including in and on healthy people. Exposure to them is unavoidable and constant. Intestinal parasites come in many forms, and they can cause a wide range of health problems. Some of the most common are amoebas, *Giardia*, and *Cryptosporidium*. These are single-celled microscopic organisms called protozoa (like *Babesia*, which are spread by tick bites). Small or large, parasites feed off of you. The larger worm parasites release eggs that can migrate throughout your body and cause many symptoms for which they are unlikely to ever be considered in diagnosis. *Giardia* is a vile parasite that is transmitted mostly through water for both drinking and swimming. Unfortunately chlorine does not kill it! Sorry dog owners, but *Giardia* (as well as colon bacteria) can be transmitted from kissing your pets (you know where else they kiss!). It is complete urban legend that a dog's mouth is clean. Improperly cooked or properly washed foods contain Giardia.

Why so much talk about *Giardia*? The obsession with Lyme *Borrelia*, in my experience has been the road to ruin for so many people. *Giardia* is a perfect example of a parasite that can cause joint and muscle pain, psychiatric problems, allergies, chronic fatigue, and general immune system impairment. Does this sound familiar? The Lyme ignorant physicians who do not acknowledge their patients' symptoms as being from tick-borne illness may have a point, but for the wrong reasons. The droves of parasitic life forms that commonly inhabit our bodies, upon the tick-borne assault of Lyme *Borrelia* and co-infections have a golden opportunity to flourish due to a disrupted immune system. There is no shortage of credible published academic research that documents the significance of numerous *other* parasitic organisms—all of which have the potential to cause Lyme symptoms and/or the damage of leaky gut. The human immune system is dependent upon intestinal health. This is no revelation, nor is it disputed by any scientific factions. It is also undisputed that various FDA-approved medications can irritate the lining of the intestines. Some popular over-the-counter pain medications could directly cause leaky gut—paving the way for parasites to make it worse and hasten the invasion.

How to Fix Leaky Gut Syndrome...

There is little medical agreement on what to do for leaky gut. In this book, I represent evaluation and treatment methods simply as *my* way of helping people get better. Addressing cause factors is always the focus. I do not attempt to treat leaky gut. I have no specific protocol or standard plan. Each patient requires different treatment. It does however, always revolve around bio-energetic support to help people heal themselves from chronic infection and toxicity. Knowing what does NOT need to be done is sometimes the highest hurdle to jump over.

Gluten Free is NOT All
It's Cracked Up to Be!

I have treated countless patients who were previously advised to eat a gluten-free diet, but experienced little or no improvement (and a lot of inconvenience). In case you have not been exposed to gluten mania, gluten is a protein from wheat, to which some people are allergic or sensitive. Savvy marketers have been steadily capitalizing on expanded public awareness of gluten. Going gluten-free certainly helps many people, but I think its significance is grossly exaggerated. The apparent rise in gluten intolerance and many food allergies seem to me to be the repercussions of escalating chronic infection and toxicity, in part precipitated by decades of antibiotic misuses and abuse.

Reducing sugars, starches, and grains in general is likely a good idea for shrinking the expanded openings of the intestinal lining. Some suggest it is the key to repairing leaky gut, but I emphatically disagree. Overcoming the chronic infection that causes it in the first place is top priority! I am an ardent advocate and teacher of whole foods nutrition, however it has not been the key to my patients' recovery from tick-triggered illness. Quite frankly, restricted diets concern me. If we make eating *more* complicated, it can cause even more stress and heartache. Many a patient has breathed a sigh of relief when informed that no special diet was required for success.

Probiotic Supplementation

I do indeed advocate probiotic supplementation (for some, but not *all* patients) to help restore beneficial bacteria to the gastrointestinal tract. This is particularly important for those patients who have had extensive antibiotic treatment. I have personally and professionally tried various probiotic supplements, but have been happiest with those cultured from *human* micro-flora. I now exclusively use the HMF line of probiotics from Genestra/Seroyal. Most brands are cultured from cattle-based sources which is fine, but not likely as readily utilized by the human body. Although replacing "friendly" bacteria is a useful strategy for improving destroyed immune function, it is a tiny component leading to my patients' recovery. The majority of all new patients have been taking probiotics for quite some time prior to entering the Liebell Clinic. Some people do not need them, and for others they can even be harmful. One must not assume they are beneficial.

Core Biting Back Principle: When the intestinal lining is inflamed and "leaky," bacteria and fungi, and other parasites can pass infection to anywhere else in your body, including your *brain*. This is **NOT** something that can be fixed simply with probiotic supplements!

Excessive Enzyme Envy

Perhaps you have already implemented enzyme supplementation. Many a patient has reported to me having futilely spent thousands of dollars over many years on enzymes, Digestive enzymes are certainly important for proper breakdown of food. Raw foods including vegetables, nuts, seeds, and fruits are rich in them. Cooking food does destroy them. Many thoughtful and effective practitioners have helped patients by encouraging patients to increase enzymes. This may improve intestinal health. However, it does not likely shrink the leaky gut. Unless the immune system is effectively dealing with parasitic life forms, the leaky gut will continue to leak, and the circle of dysfunction will continue. My advice is always to obtain nutrients from whole foods rather than questionable and expensive pills. Eat more raw vegetables and fruits. Use a blender and/or a juicer to naturally supplement your diet if you are looking for more enzymes. You don't need a doctoral degree in biochemistry if you eat whole foods!

111

There are some laboratories from which doctors can order tests that provide evidence for leaky gut. I consider it a questionable investment, since results of such rarely, if ever guide my patients and me towards better results. Quite frankly, it is a very reasonably safe assumption that anybody that enters my clinic has a leaky gut! Chronic infection and overuse of antibiotics and anti-inflammatory drugs causes openings of the intestines to expand. This increased permeability or "leaky gut" is the root of a heinous cycle that involves allergy, toxicity, liver dysfunction, and a long list of symptoms that lead the patient down a dark chasm of misdiagnosis and masking of symptoms with drugs.

Chapter 15

Why Herbal Medicine Is *Not* **Part of the Equation**

Some practitioners staunchly reject Western medicine and turn to herbal medicine—Teasel root, cat's claw, and Samento to name a few commonly utilized. In some cases, the patient suffers the burden of self-treatment with complicated herbal protocols rather than an expert doctor's guidance.

When herbs can fail to restore health to victims of tick-triggered illness, it is often for the *same* reasons antibiotics fail. The chemicals in herbs are unlikely to cross the **blood-brain-barrier.** This is the filtration system of your blood vessels that keeps harmful substances out of your brain. Antibiotics are mostly unable to cross the blood-brain-barrier, which is one of several reasons why Lyme and other infections come back with a vengeance. When pathogens and parasites exist in your brain, all the drugs in the world won't get rid of them. Your immune system must do the job! Herbal drugs act in basically the same manner as pharmaceutical medicines—they *chemically* affect the body to suppress symptoms. Herbal medicine certainly has its place in the health care of the world. I have professional access to herbs for my patients, but I will not use them for various reasons.

Herbs are *complex and concentrated* substances. Herbal plant extractions are the raw forms of many prescription medications, thus our bodies may process them in the same manner. Whether it's pharmaceutical or herbal medicine, your body must break down the chemical substances of both through digestion in order to absorb them before our cells can use them. Why is this important? It is *very* important… because your body requires <u>energy</u> to accomplish this. If you are sick and low on energy, this is bad. The secret to my patients' success in overcoming chronic tick-triggered illness is *minimal* intervention or interference. We want your body to have the *smallest* amount of complication. It's a less-is-more (done correctly) philosophy. We want MAXIMUM energy allocated by your body—to fight off all of the various parasitic and abnormal life forms that have overwhelmed it.

Safety and Regulation of Herbal Products

Herbal medicines have poor, if any government regulation. DNA tests show that many herbal supplements do not contain what they claim on the label. Lots of herbs come from China or India, where they use unregulated pesticides and other atrocious chemicals. Herbs can have side effects and drug interactions, just like any prescription or over-the-counter medication. Americans spend an estimated $5 billion a year on herbal supplements. It is wise to think of herbal medications as pharmaceutical drugs, and use them accordingly. Conventional medications are often based upon chemicals found in herbs. It is trouble enough that many FDA-approved drugs have unknown mechanisms of action, and are of doubtful quality, effectiveness, and safety. Herbal medicines pose risks that I am not willing to have my patients take. Many of them are still taking prescription medications, which can absolutely have harmful interactions with herbs.

Doctors who distinguish themselves as integrative or functional medicine practitioners seem more open-minded or "natural" because they prescribe herbs and nutritional supplements in addition to antibiotics. In my opinion, "playing Russian roulette" with unregulated herbal medications is risky, and most importantly, in my experience unnecessary. The designation of herbal or "natural" hardly equates automatically with safety. Herbs should be used with great caution and knowledge. It is

114

horrifying enough that *government-regulated* medicine is one of the leading causes of death in the United States. I do not utilize herbs in my practice. I wouldn't risk my own family's health, nor would I risk yours! Quite frankly, most of my patients had already tried herbs, and did not get well. Why reproduce what has previously failed? Trying to target and kill every microbe in your body with "natural" herbal medicines makes no more sense than attempting to do so with pharmaceuticals. If your immune system is not functioning better—if the avenues of detoxification and drainage are not improved, better health is not achieved.

Chapter 16

The "More is Better" Betrayal

Doing *more* types of treatment will generally be *less* effective, more confusing, complicated, and challenging. In my experience, the hardest part in helping sufferers of tick-triggered illness is encouraging them to give up some of their disempowering beliefs about Lyme disease, medicine, and health. Patients tend to over-think and overdo. Most have become accustomed to having multiple interventions, in greater quantities, with more frequent usage. The toughest challenge in guiding victims of Lyme disease victims towards wellness is convincing them that less is more (done correctly)!

In my experience, those who resist the temptation to overtax their bodies with complex regimens get the best results. This is not a matter of ego or conceit, but rather your best chances at success—and to save you money. Most people have arrived at my office having spent indecent amounts of money on all kinds of evaluation and treatment, in a futile attempt to recover from chronic illness and pain. I have professional access to nearly any nutritional, herbal, or other health product or device, which I could easily sell for a substantial profit. However, I have not seen these further my patients' progress. In fact, it has been quite the opposite. Those individuals, who insist on taking piles of vitamins, herbs, oils, detoxification products, antibiotics, and other products, do not respond as well.

We want the *gentlest* possible treatment—so your body can allocate its energies toward rejuvenation and repair, rather than the chore of breaking down and assimilating chemicals and other physical components of vitamins, minerals, herbs, and pharmaceutical medicines. We do not want to stress your body with a greater workload, nor do we want to stress your *wallet* with unnecessary expenses. Neither will propel you any faster or better towards results. You will learn more in the section on the *Bio-energetic Individual Treatment Equation.* Its design is such that it adds nothing challenging for your body to process, leaving maximum energy for your body's own natural systems to get to work at fighting the chronic infectious agents, eliminating toxins, and repairing damaged tissues as much as possible.

> ## *"It is useless to do with more what can be done with less."*
> - William of Ockham, English philosopher (1288-1347)

Ockham's Razor is the principle that suggests the simplest explanation of a phenomenon is most likely to be correct. This idea was not original to William of Ockham. It can be found in the works of Aristotle and others. Not everybody agrees with the concept of minimal intervention for maximum effect, nor would it apply to every situation. Ockham's suggestion was that simplicity minimizes mistakes. The more things you do to try to help—the more you risk *failure.*

The BITE is simple, yet sophisticated. It is safe, specific, and successful. Minimal but magnificent. Those patients who comply with this approach achieve the best results. My best advice is to apply the system, and not complicate matters with Lyme protocols and other methods you have come to believe are necessary. Evaluate the *Bio-Energetic Individual Treatment Equation's* results based on it alone. Why spend more money on treatments that don't improve your outcome? Whether it's the advice of Aristotle, William of Ockham, Albert Einstein, or Liebell—simple is often best.

"Nothing in the world makes people so afraid as the influence of independent-minded people." – Albert Einstein, 1879-1955

Chapter 17

Who Are The True Health Authorities?

In mathematics, there may be numerous ways to arrive at a solution to a problem. The same applies to health care. There are many treatments, techniques, systems, philosophies, sciences, and arts that can enable recovery from illness or injury, and/or prevention and health maintenance. Unfortunately, in America, conventional Western medicine has been positioned, marketed, and politicized as *the* model of health care. Medical doctors (MDs) are perceived as the ultimate unopposable authorities. Any other system or approach outside of drugs, surgery, or physical therapy is mockingly classified as alternative medicine. The *American Medical Association* is a doctors' *lobbyist* organization that has ingrained this as public opinion. The AMA was not formed for patient advocacy or health care, but rather the business needs of doctors. Many excellent books and articles have been written to cover this subject.

The masses complain about the ruthless and rich pharmaceutical companies. Medical error is currently among the leading causes of death in America. We know drugs rarely address the *causes* of the problems for which they are designed to treat. Cancer is still on the rise. Heart disease is still on the rise. The same is true for diabetes. Lyme disease has <u>always</u> been a problem but was not always officially recognized. We have more chronic illness than ever before. Yet the public still *reveres* the drug-based medical establishment as the "authorities." The public is afraid to fully accept the valuable contributions of doctors from around the globe, who practice different methods—safe and natural holistic methods. There is still a perception that we are a bunch of crazy conspiracy theorists, tree huggers, pseudo-scientists, hippies, crystal-wavers, snake oil salesmen, and kooks. NO! Many natural health methods are scientific, safe, and highly effective. Since conventional medicine clearly cannot get their act together for handling tick-triggered illness and the expanding chronic disease dilemma, I say let's leave it to HEALTH experts—not disease management experts.

People are petrified to confront their doctors because they are scared they will be dismissed as patients, and have to find another practice that accepts new patients. Mainstream doctors notoriously trash and bash *natural* methods, causing the public to be highly skeptical. We are constantly bombarded with a million questions about how they work, and their safety. My question is where is the scrutiny for *mainstream* medicine? Where's the *skepticism?* Throughout the history of modern medicine, various "wonder drugs" have proven to be disastrous. The drug thalidomide for example, was hailed by the health authorities to provide safe and sound sleep as well as relief for morning sickness of pregnancy. It was catastrophically responsible for over 10,000 infant birth defects and 5,000 deaths worldwide. The precise mechanism of action for thalidomide is still unknown.

Do you think your doctor can explain the biochemistry and mechanism of action in the body for the antibiotic, *doxycycline?* I think it is revolting that doctors are permitted to keep patients on a revolving door of doxycycline and other antibiotics for *years*. Are those doctors heroes just because they "believe in" chronic Lyme disease? Big deal! We're talking about a debilitating disease here—not the tooth fairy! All doctors (regardless of specialty) should be knowledgeable about tick-borne infection. I do not think any doctors (including myself) deserve any special credit or praise for accepting reality. For those fortunate patients, who have been able to merely take doxycycline, and have an effective enough immune system to finish the job, and get well… I am thrilled. My commentary is designed for the massive population of people, who suffer pain and illness within the conventional medical system, which has left them ravaged with complex problems—that will not, and cannot be cured with a *pill*. I never intended to have anything to do with Lyme disease. I became deeply involved with it as a result of my wife, Sheila's experience, and the coincidental study of the methods that ultimately enabled her recovery. I had a successful chiropractic practice for a long time, and I was hardly looking to complicate my life. It became a calling and a responsibility to provide critically-needed help for others too.

No individual doctor or organization can boast the title of the foremost or all-knowing authority on Lyme disease or for that matter, any other aspect of human health and medical treatment. I am no exception to the rule. In fact, I am appalled by the distinction of Lyme literate doctor—for any physician! Are there flu-literate medical doctors? What about neck pain-literate chiropractors, cavity-literate dentists, bunion-literate podiatrists, or cataract-literate optometrists? Sarcastic and silly as my challenge may sound, it is quite serious. Shouldn't *all* doctors be literate in a disease that can affect any organ or system in the body? Would you think it odd if you went to a physician who was not at least familiar, let alone have some working knowledge about strep throat, bronchitis, broken bones, dental cavities, or dozens of other common ailments? It would certainly be unacceptable. Let's stop lavishly praising doctors for doing what should be expected and required. It would be more appropriate to refer to Lyme-ignorant doctors, who put blinders on to a major cause of illness throughout the world.

If the *National Institutes of Health* ever comes knocking on my door to offer me a huge research grant to conduct a study to document and publish the effectiveness of the *Bio-energetic Individual Treatment Equation*© I will be ready and eager to participate. But I'm not holding my breath! And I must emphatically repeat over and over that I make no medical claims to treat or cure any particular disease. My evidence is my patients' dramatic improvements, documented by the patients themselves.

An Extremely Decent Proposal

Perhaps someday a health organization, university, or philanthropic person or entity will be willing to fund a study of the BITE. I embrace the challenge to personally take on a large sample of patients from whom all other medical care has failed—and put it to the test. Let us track the changes for each patient over the course of one year. The costs of such a study would be miniscule in comparison to most health care research projects. The lives that would be changed without the need of a single drug would more than justify the expense. If treatment were funded such that no costs were involved for patients, there would likely be no shortage of volunteers.

I would propose the following research scenario:

Three groups of patients with similar medical history profiles of chronic tick-triggered illness would be randomly segregated. The control group would receive BITE evaluation, but no treatment. The placebo group would receive BITE evaluation, including sham auricular therapy, which would be easily applied without patient knowledge of simulation. They would then receive placebo bio-energetic support supplements, which would be merely solutions of water and alcohol, with no encoded information imprints embedded. The third group would receive authentic evaluation, auricular therapy treatment and bio-energetic supplementation. All groups would be re-evaluated as per standard BITE protocol every two months, and data recorded.

The double-bind control study is considered the standard scientific research model. However, I must ponder the ethical conundrum of giving realistic hope to a group of sick and suffering people who are desperate for help, knowing only a maximum of one third of them could receive benefit. Patients who seek my care have *already* suffered for years—failing to improve their health through implementing various treatment approaches and spending outlandish sums of money. I have no doubt that sham treatments would be ineffective. Unless there is an academic research requirement for a control and placebo group, my preference would be to bypass these research parameters, and simply provide the holistic supportive treatment to all participants in the study. The agent of cure is still the human immune system, which does not need to be proven in the manner of a drug.

Even though all participant could receive proper treatment at the end of the study, I would hate to see two thirds of study participants receive no health improvement for an entire year, and suffer needlessly. My empathetic doctor's brain is partial to proving a point by helping as many people as possible, and letting that speak for the effectiveness of this wellness based approach.

Should anybody have criticism of the *Bio-energetic Individual Treatment Equation©* I will be armed and ready to discuss it publicly and through the media. There is an endless sea of controversial, questionable, and downright dangerous medical procedures. Many have come and gone already. Others escape scrutiny until enough carnage becomes publicized. Every day, scientists reveal that various medical tests and treatments need to be re-evaluated, revamped, and in many cases removed. They call it reversal when scientific knowledge mandates the change. Medical journals report reversals of hundreds of practices as decades go by. What was once firmly established as the standard of treatment becomes dangerous or antiquated. Consider the arthritis drug Vioxx, which was found to be responsible for over 60,000 deaths before being discontinued in 2004. Medical research is fraught with conflicts of interest too. Money drives the result, regardless of safety.

We can go on and on about the dangers of conventional medical practices. I could dig up and quote study after study that proves the point. America spends the most on health care, but we cannot boast the best *health* as a result. Not by a long shot. Chronic illness is out of control, and medical error is one of the leading causes of death—hundreds of thousands alone due to pharmaceutical medication. Our conventional medical system rarely provides health care. It delivers disease *management*—obscenely profitable drug-based treatment that mostly maintains illness.

My treatment has not, and will not harm anybody. It has produced extraordinary results for people who had nowhere else to turn. It requires no defense or justification. The fact that mainstream medicine is unlikely to ever take it seriously is irrelevant. Naysayers can blab on and on until they're blue in the face about why it *couldn't* work, doesn't work, or that results are just the placebo effect. Both my grateful patients and I will cheerfully and humbly reply, we don't care what they think!

There are various books and articles out there that are designed to scare the public away from so-called alternative medicine. Their premise is that there can be only one king in the castle to rule health care. Although this is terrible—it works both ways. There is a lot of complete and utter garbage out there in the alternative medicine field, although nowhere near approaching conventional Western medicine, where the death toll is proof positive. Despite its faults, Western medicine as a whole should be applauded, and certainly not avoided. That would be foolish. The advances in health care that have drastically improved the quality of human life cannot be underestimated. This does not however, give Western medicine a free pass to do whatever it wants without scrutiny. No medical system is perfect.

Many books and articles have been written for the explicit purpose of discrediting alternative medicine. One argument is that alternative medicine is used in countries where Western medications are scarce because it's all they've got. They wish they had "real medicine." This of course does not hold water considering that Germany is the birthplace of homeopathy, where it has been used continuously for over 200 years. The Chinese have not abandoned acupuncture either.

Critics of natural health methods tend to argue that we holistic doctors are using unproven or pseudoscientific methods. The assumption that conventional medical establishment is the judge and jury on what constitutes science is highly debatable. If we consider that over 100,000 people die every year from supposedly correctly prescribed drugs, it alone gives us reason to question their authority. I can certainly state with pride that my treatment, which naturally guides people towards healing from within, is not going to kill anybody! Implementing the *Bio-energetic Individual Treatment Equation*© has not destroyed anybody's gut bacteria, caused rapid die-off toxic side effects, nor has it caused anybody to become addicted to controlled poisons.

Somewhere along the line, the term, alternative medicine was created to describe treatment methods that do not conform to the current establishment's traditions. Odd isn't it that acupuncture, and other highly effective and safe, natural treatments that long preceded pharmaceutical medicine are referred to as alternative? Personally, I prefer the term natural and holistic health care. It implies neither inferiority nor superiority to conventional drugs or surgery.

124

Throughout every era of human history, the controlling authorities of the time have professed to possess all of the knowledge. New ideas are customarily considered radical, crazy, or subversive. The famous German philosopher, Schopenhauer (1788 – 1860) once said, "All truth passes through three stages. First, it is ridiculed. Second, it is violently opposed. Third, it is accepted as being self-evident." Statistically, there is substantial motivation to question who the health authorities really are. The trends for chronic illness have worsened progressively, despite advancements in scientific knowledge and technology. More than half of all Americans suffer from one or more chronic illnesses!

The Wellness Model of Health Care vs. the Disease Model

An ounce of prevention is worth a pound of cure. It is a nice sentiment. Everybody knows it's true, just like the Golden Rule. But to what degree is the adage's principle practically applied? Remarkably, the answer appears to be infrequently. In fact, insurance companies don't pay for true health care—the promotion of wellness and the prevention of illness. They pay for diagnosis and treating the effects of disease! Health support vs. disease treatment—the two are as different as night and day. Overhauling a toxic diet, exercise, and other healthful practices promote *wellness* for a person suffering cardiovascular disease, high blood pressure, and other obesity-related problems. Statin drugs, blood pressure pills, and other heart medications treat symptoms of *disease*.

We see modern doctors using outdated techniques. The world has changed tremendously, but conventional Western medical philosophy and its associated methods have remained stagnant. The symptoms you're struggling to eradicate have grown *increasingly immune* to the conventional medical approach. In

125

today's over-medicated, toxic world, the same old techniques for battling diseases (not just Lyme) may still work, *but not nearly as well as they used to*. This is why most so many people are suffering pain and illness. This trend will inevitably continue, as bacteria and other parasitic life forms grow *increasingly immune* to an ever-rising flood of the same tired, overworked antibiotic-centered approach.

Functional medicine: a New Twist on an Old Idea?

A faction of doctors has recently arrived on the scene boasting the evolution of a *new* concept called functional medicine. Their startling revelation is that doctors should focus on the individual patient, and the causes and mechanisms of disease within each person as a whole. The contrary approach is the rigid categorization, diagnosis, and treatment of named illnesses. Doctors trained in functional medicine tout their focus on *why* symptoms are occurring and what their root causes are. They criticize their conventional Western medicine colleagues' focus on what disease a person has.

I couldn't agree with their philosophy more, but seriously... is this a *new* idea? I find this "specialty" to be simultaneously encouraging, insulting, pompous, and puzzling. It appears to me that these doctors have deceptively disguised themselves—assuming a pretentious new identity. The functional medicine approach is precisely what many health professionals worldwide been unconscionably *vilified* for practicing for ages. **It is called holistic health care!** Chiropractors, acupuncturists, naturopaths, homeopaths, osteopaths, and other outstanding practitioners suffering the indignity of the obnoxious label, alternative medicine, have adopted this humane philosophy and practice for centuries! And we have done so despite violent attack and persecution at the hands of *American Medical*

126

Association. Now, a few conventionally-trained physicians, who have recently become enlightened to the shortcomings of their own system (and perhaps are keenly aware of the public's disenchantment with mainstream medicine) are proudly proclaiming the merits of *our* long-coveted wellness principles. Shamelessly giving a fancy new title to the philosophy, art, and science of holistic medicine is hardly impressive to me. They seem to be taking credit for the vital principles of health care that we holistic and natural practitioners have *always* utilized.

A Touch of the "Golden Rule" in Medicine?

Another attribute proclaimed by the functional medicine faction is showing greater compassion and interest, and spending more time with the patient than the conventional provider. This includes much more detail and history beyond the symptoms of your chief medical complaint. But wait... there's more! Functional medicine doctors will also construct a treatment plan that includes health lifestyle changes including diet and exercise, stress management, reducing exposure to toxins, and other factors. The functional medicine approach can include prescription drugs, nutritional supplements, detoxification regimens, and herbal medicines too. The doctor plays an active role as a health coach, rather than merely a prescription writer. ***Isn't this what doctors are supposed to do?***

Practitioners of the "new" functional medicine are proud to report that unlike their conventional colleagues, they address the underlying causes of disease, and that they focus on multiple systems of the body. They are staking claim to the breakthrough concept of patient-centered focus—shifting away from the conventional *disease*-oriented focus. Their newly- found philosophy is addressing the whole person, and to take a more active and personalized role in the patient's health. Hello... am I the only one seeing through this smoke screen? I recently

127

participated in an online medical conference focusing on autoimmune disease. The presenters arrogantly gushed about functional medicine like they just invented the wheel! I cringed at the doctors boasting that they are looking at the body in a whole new way—a wellness approach. The revelation is that doctors must look at more than pathology—with the understanding that disease is not a phenomenon that can be isolated as the same in each individual. One must consider genetic predispositions, metabolic capacity, sleep cycles, past injury, and other individual components of the person, not just a disease.

Once again, this describes the principles of holistic medicine practiced for hundreds, or like in the case of acupuncture, thousands of years! Are we supposed to be monumentally impressed now that a few conventionally-educated medical doctors have finally opened up to what their perceived *inferior* practitioners have done all along? It is not eye-opening that every patient has unique needs, which may require different treatments, either separately or simultaneously. The fact that conventional medications and diagnostic tests may be *integrated* into the long-established holistic equation does not constitute a new way of thinking! Despite these indiscretions, these are *excellent doctors*, who in my opinion are a cut above the rest. I applaud them for recognizing that disease is neither the beginning nor the end point. They acknowledge it as a process of development that may not be discovered until symptoms or physical changes are revealed to indicate an illness. These physicians grasp the importance of taking a different approach for treating chronic pain and illness from that of acute illness. They finally comprehend that there is more to health care than giving a patient a named condition, which is treated as the entity rather than the patient as a whole. Praise them for their recent enlightenment and newly found expertise, which will benefit the public tremendously. My criticism is their hijacking of the long-utilized principles and practices of holistic practitioners around the world, and staking a claim to them as their discovery or invention.

I am aware that there are various doctors who say their treatments cure Lyme disease. I, on the other hand, do not make such a claim. What I do say is that *the human immune system* is capable of fighting of Lyme *Borrelia* bacteria, as well as thousands of other infectious microorganisms. And I am very proud to have proven with case after case, the ability to support restoration of normal function of sick and suffering people—regardless of a confirmed Lyme (or other) diagnosis. That's what true healing, authentic wellness care, and scientific energy medicine are all about.

Please do not misconstrue my detailed explanations of the mechanisms of antibiotics, herbs, diets, detoxification, Rife machines, etc., as bashing the competition. It is not. In fact, I applaud anybody and any method that delivers successful *results*. However, let me clarify that my definition of success may differ from that of other doctors (and some patients). I view successful results as being when a person, who has long suffered pain and illness, recovers *without* drugs masking or suppressing their symptoms. Success is when a person becomes truly healthier and functional.

It's a free country. You *should* consider any of the treatments found across the Internet and in the offices of those proclaiming themselves Lyme specialists. But get all the facts about those methods too. Put them all to the same level of scrutiny. Lyme disease may not be the conspiracy theory condition it has been portrayed to be. It may simply be one of the thousands of health issues that are the consequence of exploitation of medical technology, greed, politics, and a lost focus on what health really is, and how it can be achieved. You have the free will and the freedom to choose the health care methods that appeal to you. Authorities are typically self-appointed. My expertise is in natural health, wellness, and pain relief. However, I am not *against* anything that reduces human suffering, provided that long-term consequences are not sacrificed for short-term or instant gratification. My patients can assure you that getting well is a *marathon... not a sprint.* But oh, what a worthwhile journey the marathon is!

"I sought treatment by several doctors prior to seeing Dr. Liebell. I saw my internist, who does not believe that Lyme disease was prevalent in our area, a neurologist, who had never treated Lyme disease, but was very willing to do research and provided me with the necessary antibiotics. I also saw a rheumatologist who would not diagnose Lyme disease, prescribed more cortisone and keep insisting the swollen hand was inflammation.

The benefits from the treatments were almost immediate relief from the swelling and pain. After two weeks, I was able to use my hand again and resume a good sleeping pattern at night. The swelling had endured for three very painful months and then after the treatment began, my hand gradually returned to normalcy. I continue to follow up with Dr. Liebell at two month intervals just to tweak my program and keep my good health in progress. Many of the tinctures are no longer necessary, but we safeguard my health by adjusting to protect against any other health issues that occur." - Gerard N. - Hertford, North Carolina, 2013

Part Four:

The Bio-energetic Individual Treatment Equation

The art of healing comes from nature, not from the physician.
Therefore the physician must start from nature, with an open mind.

- Paracelsus

(Renaissance physician, founder of medical toxicology)

Chapter 18

Immune System 101

A Simple Explanation of Your Body's Inborn Defense System… and Why it is Capable of Overcoming Tick-Triggered Illness

We all harbor viruses, bacteria, fungi, and other assorted pathogens and parasites in our bodies—but not everybody suffers illnesses. A healthy immune system can usually handle the situation. Like it or not, our bodies are *normally* loaded full of organisms that could cause disease. The key is how well each body manages them to maintain a healthy balance and prevent them from overwhelming the system. In fact, it is virtually impossible to be alive and not be carrying potentially pathogenic organisms.

Your own body is what holds the key to overcoming illness due to infection. If your body's natural systems are not better… <u>you</u> are not better! The *Bio-energetic Individual Treatment Equation*© is all about supporting the restoration of normal body function. Human immune systems have been capably fighting infection for as long as humans have roamed the earth. Our bodies have always been inhabited by microbes, with the immune system on the task to battle the bugs. So, what exactly is the immune system? That is the purpose of this chapter.

In my experience, those who understand a little bit about how the immune system works tend to have an easier time following through and doing what it takes to get well. There's no need for despair—this isn't going to be a college course in anatomy and physiology, and there won't be a pop quiz! I have included this information as a reference. Although I highly recommend you read it all, you won't hurt my feelings if you skip it!

Here's what it is all about:

The immune system fights against infectious microorganisms (microbes, germs) and other irritants. We call the various steps it takes the **immune response**. The parts of our great defense system include a vast network of cells, tissues, and organs that protect the body. We have several types of **white blood cells** (leukocytes), which are the chief attackers of germs. Some white blood cells "eat" the bacteria, viruses, fungi, and other invaders. Others are responsible for "remembering and recognizing" these invaders from previous exposure.

One measure of immune system function is counting the numbers of the different types of white blood cells in a sample of blood. A low white cell count can suggest various problems, including infection. The normal count should be between 4,500 and 10,000 cells per micro liter. In addition to illness, there are numerous prescription drugs that can alter white blood cell counts. The CD57 blood test can be a useful indicator of a troubled immune system.

Antigens and Antibodies

We call a foreign substance that invades and irritates the body an **antigen**. Your body "recognizes" that specific proteins from viruses, bacteria, fungi, etc. are not human cells. The immune system develops **antibodies**, which are specialized proteins that provide the "memory" for the body to signal a defense, should future exposure of the germs take place. That's what immunity is all about! But memory isn't enough; there must be a system of attack. That's what white blood cells known as **T-cells** do. They are produced by your **thymus gland** located near your heart. A healthy **spleen** acts as a filter of foreign cells, and thus plays an important role of immunity. Those who have had their spleen removed tend to get sick more often.

Types of Immunity

When you are born, you already have some immune system defense capability. This is called **innate immunity**. Your first line of defense against germs also includes your skin, as well as the lining of your nose, throat, and gastrointestinal system. If a virus, bacteria, or other microbe gets past this wall, it's up to your white blood cells to launch their attack.

We also have immunity that develops throughout our lives. Exposure to germs triggers this protective immune response. There are some diseases that once you've had them, you are protected against future infection. The intention of immunization through vaccination is to create controlled exposure to a *weakened* form of a particular microorganism, which provokes an ongoing immune response of protection against the actual infection, if encountered. In other words, a tiny amount of the disease protein is injected so the immune system will "recognize" and deal with the real thing, should it come along—without causing the actual disease in the process.

Why Some People Don't Get Sick

Life is not fair. We are all born with different strengths and weaknesses, as well as aptitudes and abilities. For some people, math comes easily, but for others it is a struggle. The same is true for music, art, or sports. Immunity and health are no different. Genetics do play a role, but I am certain they are blamed too much. Some people are impervious to certain illnesses. They seem to have an impenetrable wall of defense against specific viruses, for example. Do you know somebody who never gets the flu or catches cold, even when the bug is going around? A sick person could cough right in his or her face, but no illness develops. Not fair, is it?

I'll bet you know somebody who says they don't get mosquito bites. Maybe he or she is an outdoorsy type, who boasts being

134

bitten by ticks thousands of times, without the slightest Lyme disease symptom ever experienced. How can this be? Don't ticks spread Lyme disease? Don't mosquitoes spread viruses? Yes, they do, but that doesn't mean the person bitten will be affected! The reason some people are affected, while others are not is the strength and abilities of each individual's <u>immune system</u>.

What Goes Wrong?

Nobody is perfect, and neither is anybody's immune system. Everyone has a breaking point. When your body becomes overwhelmed by any stress, it can become disabled in its power to defend itself. If you recall from the chapter on antibiotics, "superbugs" can "outwit" an unhealthy immune system. And when one's immune system becomes interfered with from one source, it can become an easy target for all kinds of other germs.

"Party Time" for the Microbes

Numerous viruses are responsible for more of the problems Lyme victims suffer than the *Borrelia* bacteria. Lyme bacteria are without a doubt, capable of ravaging one's immune system. What this does is open the door for every opportunistic pathogen and parasite to wreak havoc on your body. Viruses can exist in our bodies for decades, even if they're not reproducing enough to directly cause illness. Consider the case of chicken pox and shingles. One could have chicken pox as a child, recover, and have its causative *Varicella zoster* virus lay dormant for 50 or 60 years. Then, in a moment of immune system interference (usually due to another illness) it can come out of hibernation and "gratefully" punish its fragile host with the often excruciating shingles nerve pain!

Don't forget that viruses can be spread from person-to-person without any symptoms of obvious illness developing. Consider HIV and AIDS. An HIV positive person may not develop the disease, but could spread it to somebody who ultimately does. And what is AIDS? It is *Acquired Immune Deficiency Syndrome*. The name depicts the destruction of the immune system's ability to do its job. The AIDS victim develops many illnesses, many of which are due to various other germs—not the HIV itself. These can include deadly infections from bacteria, other viruses, and parasites of all kinds. A poorly functioning immune system can create a breeding ground for fungal disease. I'm not just talking about *Candida* (yeast infection), which is the least of your problems. There are *hundreds* of species of fungi that cause disease. The toxins released by some fungi are among the most cancer-causing substances known!

Typhoid Mary

In 1907, Mary Mallon, a cook from Ireland, did not think it was necessary to wash her hands. She was a healthy carrier of the bacterium, *Salmonella typhi*. She had what is known as a subclinical infection, which she spread to dozens of Americans as Typhoid fever. "Typhoid Mary" did not clinically have Typhoid fever—but she was indeed infected. We now know that there are dozens and dozens of subclinical infections. One may be harboring various germs in one's body, without any symptoms associated with them at all. What this means is that a person can be bitten by an infectious tick, but not develop Lyme disease (or perhaps not right away)! Germs do not cause disease in every person. Immune systems are of different capabilities in each person, and that is why some people do not get sick from certain viruses, bacteria, and other pathogens, but others do. The purpose of the *Bio-energetic Individual Treatment Equation*© is to support your body's normal function so it gains the ability to fight the germs that are agents of disease via an effectively functioning immune system.

Immune Deficiency, Autoimmune, and Allergic Disorders

An infectious tick bite is not necessarily the starting point of one's illness. However, it may deliver the knock-out punch. One might have hundreds of problems brewing beneath the surface—kept in check by the immune system. Add the parasitic puncture from a wretched tick... and it's all downhill from there! New allergies develop. Thyroid gland malfunction creeps up on you. Sinusitis is now a menace. Colds and stomach viruses are now an ongoing presence. What gives? The answer is simple: your immune system got systematically hammered by a variety of sources, one of which was likely Lyme *Borrelia* bacterial infection.

Toxic chemicals are a fact of life, more so than any time in human history. Our alleged protector, the *U.S. Food and Drug Administration* (FDA) has allowed chemical poisons (toxins) to exist in countless industries. They make their way into our bodies by too many routes to mention. Toxins can disorient or disable the immune system. This paves the way for germs to harm us even more. Modern medical technology cannot compensate for our bodies being overwhelmed by toxins that did not exist thousands of years ago. Our ancestors had other dangers, but they never had to deal with modern chemical stress. It is possible that toxins alone have made us humans more susceptible to disease than ever before. I believe that in a way, it is harder to stay healthy now—more than any time in our history. One might think it would be easier. Guess again!

Disease doesn't just show up; everything has causes. It may be the case that disruption of the immune system (by various means) is the ultimate cause of all chronic illness. It has been observed for years that autoimmune conditions develop after viral or bacterial infections. These disorders often have the same symptoms as active infection. This is why many Lyme victims will insist they're still infected, and seek more antibiotics! In cases of cancer, the immune system may fail to "recognize" the cancer cells as being an enemy. The cells may not be different enough from healthy human cells to warrant an attack from the white blood cells. Or the individual's immune response may be malfunctioning such that it cannot get the job done.

Unpleasant, but Important

To best understand the extraordinary raw power of the immune system in overcoming illness, consider what happens to a body upon *death*. This might seem obvious to say, but only a *living* person has a functioning immune system. Once a person dies, all systems cease to function. It takes only a mere matter of hours for dead body to become overrun by all kinds of parasites and pathogens. The *living* body's immune system protected it against these countless invaders. With no immune system on patrol it truly becomes party time for the microbes, as well as all kinds of insects and worms (yuck!). The parade of opportunists will completely dismantle the body down to the bone in a matter of weeks.

Life is beautiful. Perhaps with this brief, but unpleasant scenario understood, you can appreciate that your immune system performs unfathomable tasks every moment of your life— preventing its destruction. So when you have a fever, a skin irritation, a swollen joint, or any kind of inflammation, you will praise the sheer brilliance of your immune system. Every day of your life, you breathe in thousands of viruses, bacteria, and fungi from the air. Your immune system deals with them most of the time without a hitch. You eat all kinds of pathogens and parasites too, but the acids of your stomach take care of most of them.

More Parts of the Immune System

There exists a body system for which most people never give a thought, and doctors seem to hardly ever mention. It is a

138

disease-fighting, internal cleansing system that if properly supported, can massively boost your health and well-being. Did you know that you had a system of vessels (in addition to your blood vessels) that carries away and filters out poisons and waste products throughout your body? It's called the **lymphatic system**, and if you've never heard of it before, or don't know what it actually does, in a moment you'll be amazed at what it accomplishes.

The Lymphatic System is a vast network of vessels, ducts, lymph nodes and other structures that interact with every organ and tissue of your body. It is dedicated to the circulation and production of your body's disease fighting "superstars" – the white blood cells. The lymphatic system also produces immune cells called **monocytes**, as well as **plasma cells**, which produce antibodies. It also transports essential fatty acids to the blood circulatory system. Lymphatic vessels carry lymph fluid, which transports substances your body removes from its tissues. The lymphatic system is the "garbage collector" of your body. It sucks out all the junk from your organs and tissues.

A peak-functioning lymphatic system helps keep you healthy, and fights the nasty effects of aging. On the other hand, if your lymph is *not* flowing well throughout your body, the fluid becomes toxic. Your body gets bogged down by its own waste products, and can become a cesspool for infection. If toxic lymph fluid gets into your bloodstream, infection can spread anywhere in your body. Poorly moving lymph fluid is much like stagnant water. If it just sits still—it becomes polluted. Germs get locked into your lymphatic system if the fluids aren't pumping throughout the vessels freely and efficiently. This can be a factor in degenerative diseases, rapid aging and early death. This is one of the reasons lymphatic drainage is studied in the diagnosis and treatment of cancer. A fouled up lymphatic system can end up carrying cancerous cells to other parts of the body. This is called metastasis.

139

If your lymphatic system is working poorly, and your lymph nodes, which are the filters of the immune system, cannot trap and destroy the cancer cells... the lymph nodes themselves can become cancerous too. That's called Hodgkin's disease. A poorly functioning or diseased lymphatic system can result in swelling in many areas of the body, and drastically reduce your body's ability to fight infection.

Lymphatic System Support: Your lymphatic vessels need your help to move the lymph fluid throughout your body! That is because your lymphatic system does NOT have an automatic pump—unlike your cardiovascular system, which has your heart to do the job. Proper lymphatic flow requires body movement, specifically contraction of skeletal muscles. There are little lymphatic valves, which contract and relax during muscular movement. Up and down movement, performed on a mini-trampoline or rebounder is perhaps the finest way to move your lymph. Do not skimp on quality. My family will use only two brands: Bellicon (Germany) and Needak (USA).

Your Immune System and Tick-Borne Infection

Have you suffered a cold at least once in your lifetime, and perhaps a fever or two? Maybe you have dealt with a chronic cough. Your body healed itself through the magnificent awe-inspiring power of the human immune system. Hurray for your white blood cells, thymus, spleen, lymph vessels, and other members of the team. Who is to say that your immune system cannot overpower the *Borrelia* bacteria? It can, and it does. Every person who has been bitten by ticks without developing Lyme disease is proof positive. We do not need a million-dollar research grant, years of research, double-blind studies, and publication in a peer-reviewed medical journal to confirm this. The existence and function of the immune system is set in stone. With the *Bio-energetic Individual Treatment Equation*© we simply acknowledge this, and work towards supporting your body, with the intention of it coming out of hibernation. There is no medical treatment to claim direct responsibility for patients' recovery. It is purely the result of the individual's own natural body systems doing the job.

We do not treat infectious disease or any specific illness by applying the *Bio-Energetic Individual Treatment Equation*. We seek elimination of blockages to normal function and healing, and gently support normal body function. What a magnificent and simple concept it is. It is its simplicity that boggles the minds of the hyper-educated medical world. It is no great leap of faith nor is it putting *trust* in alternative medicine to give one's body the opportunity to heal itself. Conventional doctors lay claim to curing the diseases with drugs. It is a scientific fact that antibiotics *suppress* immune system function. However, when put to the test, the human immune system blows away any drug made in any laboratory! What a privilege it is for me to be blessed with the opportunity see the human body in action on a daily basis.

"When I first came to Dr. Liebell it was to discuss my lower back pain. Little did I know, he was going to be able to lessen my joint pain, piriformis syndrome, hip bursitis, fatigue, and depression, as well as heal my headaches, neck, and lower back. I had no life before Dr. Liebell. My lower back pain was so excruciating that I was on pain killers and very strong muscle relaxers, and still felt pain every day. My depression was so bad I felt life was not worth living if this is what my life was going to be like. I saw doctors for 4 years, many of them saying there was nothing wrong with me and everything I was feeling was "all in my head."

I started treatment and immediately I started feeling more energy... Dr. Liebell gave me back my life. When people see me now they are astonished that a homeopathic treatment had such a strong and positive effect on my life. I can exercise whenever I want and after work I actually have the energy to clean the house or spend time with friends. I was finally smiling because I was genuinely happy! I will keep in touch with Dr. Liebell and his office for the rest of my life." - Sarah G., Virginia Beach

141

"If you want to find the secrets of the universe, think in terms of energy, frequency and vibration." — Nikola Tesla

Chapter 19

The Subtle Signals of Bio-electric Fields:

The principles of Western medicine are still based upon the misguided notion that human beings are machines. We are not. In the science of physics, the principles set forth by Isaac Newton have long transitioned in focus to the physics of Albert Einstein, which acknowledges that energy and matter are dual expressions of the same thing. That's what his famous $E\text{-}mc^2$ is all about. The bio-energy medicine view is based upon Einstein's perspective that human beings are complex networks of energy fields that coexist with the physical cellular systems. The integration of energy medicine with chemical and physical medicine creates a truly complete system. Bio-energetic evaluations and treatment are essential. Pharmaceutical and physical medicine methods ignore the electromagnetic forces that breathe life into the mechanical machinery of living bodies. The fields of mechanical and chemical engineering do not exist without electrical engineering. It is time that biomechanics and biochemistry join up with bio-*electrical* principles.

The public currently maintains a certain discomfort with the term, *energy medicine.* This is both unfortunate and logically unfounded. *Authentic* energy medicine is not hocus pocus, new age, or woo-woo as such popular jargon might depict it. Bio-energetic medicine is the detection and correction of energetic disturbances and weaknesses in the body, utilizing various medical devices and human observations. It involves attention to vibrational frequencies including those of electricity, magnetism, heat, light, sound, gravity, pressure and mechanical energy. Treatment involves various procedures that focus on these factors to support the repair of tissues. Bio-energetic evaluations can tell us a great deal about our health—leading to safe, effective and affordable treatments from many disciplines of medicine. The working principle of bio-energetic medicine is that energy *is* the "medicine"

The "Great and Powerful" Oz Speaks Up

On November 20, 2007, Dr. Mehmet Oz, expressed that the next big frontier in medicine is energy medicine. He said so on *Oprah*, the largest stage in America. While Dr. Oz is hardly the judge and jury of what is medically acceptable—people tend to trust him. He has helped many Americans learn that pharmaceutical medicine is not their only option for health care. Another outstanding source of scientific wisdom comes from James Oschman, PhD. He is known as the world authority on the subject of energy medicine. Dr. Oschman has made great strides to educate doctors and the public. He is a biophysicist who has worked in some of the world's most prestigious labs. Dr. Oschman is the author *of Energy Medicine: The Scientific Basis,* as well as *Energy Medicine in Therapeutics and Human Performance.* These two books provide the scientific basis of energy medicine to even the most skeptical academic scientists. Dr. Oschman is a member of the Scientific Advisory Board for the *National Foundation for Alternative Medicine* in Washington, DC.

How a Resurrected "Pearl of Wisdom" From a Yale Anatomy Professor's Research Leads to Health Clues That Blood Tests <u>Miss</u>!

Life is energy. All of the cells and tissues of our bodies generate electric currents. This is an undisputed and well-established scientific fact. Various bio-energetic changes can be monitored and measured using objective energy medicine technologies. Consider the electrocardiogram (ECG), which monitors heart function. An electroencephalogram (EEG) records electrical activity in the brain nerve cells. Muscle activity can be evaluated through an electromyogram (EMG). A polygraph or lie detector is an electrical detector as well. And perhaps the most famous approaches of them all the MRI, which is an acronym for Magnetic Resonance Imaging. These are all energy medicine devices, but they are not referred to as such by mainstream doctors.

We humans are firmly acknowledged as electromagnetic beings diagnostically, but rarely so therapeutically (beyond some electrotherapies and ultrasound treatment). It is peculiar that Western medicine relies heavily on these energy medicine diagnostic technologies to *see* evidence of disease or injury in the body, yet they scoff at the idea of treatment applications that can help the body heal itself naturally.

Dr. Harold Burr (1889-1973) was *Professor Emeritus of anatomy at Yale University School of Medicine.* He published 93 scientific papers regarding the nervous system and bio-energetic phenomena over a forty-year period. He also discovered the hormone, estrogen. Dr. Burr discovered that our bodies possessed a **living electric field matrix**, which he called the "L-field."

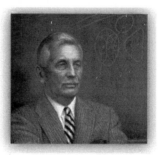

Source: www.nih.gov

Professor Burr made some phenomenal discoveries about energetic fields and their relation to health. He suggested that L-field measurements could be used to assess the general state of the body as a whole, or the effects of medical treatments. In one study he was able to detect malignant ovarian cancer by L-

144

field... before any *physical* clinical signs could be found! Burr verified his hypothesis that bio-energetic fields fluctuate around all living things, and that they are the source of all communication—before any *chemical* activity takes place. All living things are forged, organized, and guided by electro-dynamic fields. In other words, he scientifically confirmed that bio-electric fields function on a level beyond DNA to form the "blueprint" for the physical form of living things! Since abnormalities in L-field voltages can provide advanced warning of future problems—they may be equally utilized to find problems that physical and chemical tests may miss.

On the Surface of the Skin

In the late 1940s, a contemporary of Burr's, German physician Reinhold Voll, M.D. discovered that when an internal organ's function or structure was disturbed—subtle electrical changes could be detected on pinpoint areas on the surface of the skin. The Chinese had established these as *acupuncture points* thousands of years prior. Dr. Voll electrically confirmed their existence with scientific instruments. He pioneered Electro-Dermal Screening. It works by measuring electrical resistance and polarization on the skin. Voll also determined that a medication, food, supplement or any object placed in contact with a person's body, would affect electro-dermal readings. He found that merely **holding** a medication in one's hand could stimulate a measured change in the body sufficient to give insight to whether or not it might be effective—a bio-energetic response. Complementing Burr's research, Voll came to understand the great significance of energy versus matter in the scheme of health. His experiments on thousands of people revealed distinct and measurable differences in the electrodynamic natures between the healthy and sick. Instead of focusing on analysis of the chemical nature of the body, Voll's interest was energetic.

As you will learn soon, these concepts form the foundation of the *Bio-energetic Individualized Treatment Equation*. You have been raised with the bio-*chemical* model of medicine—so it may take some time to fully grasp bio-energetics. Conceptualizing or visualizing L-fields might seem troublesome. However, according to Harold Burr, there is nothing *mysterious* about living electric fields. In his 1972 book, *Blueprint for Immortality*, Burr described the school science class experiment, where iron filings

are scattered on a card held over a magnet. The filings arrange themselves in the pattern of the lines of force from the magnetic field. If the filings are discarded, and new ones are scattered on the

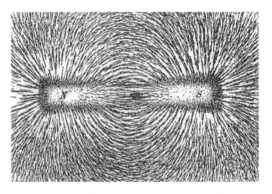

card—the same pattern emerges. In the human body, cells are constantly damaged and rebuilt from the raw materials of the foods we eat. It is the living electric fields that guide cellular reconstruction. All of your body's proteins renew every six months. Some organs and tissues do so even more frequently. Burr pointed out that if you see a friend whom you haven't seen in six months, you're not seeing the same face—but the "blueprint" of the living electric fields dictate that the new cells rebuild themselves exactly the same!

Ahead of His Time... But Now Hope for Lyme

How accurate Dr. Burr was when he predicted that extensive application of living electric fields in medicine would not be quickly embraced. He felt that since modern instruments were available, there was no good technical reason why it should take

146

doctors so long to show interest. He wasn't naïve; he knew his work was well ahead of its time. He pointed out that electrocardiogram techniques took over thirty years to become medically useful. The professor was able to foresee the link between physics, chemistry, and biology, which was validated scientifically with applications of ECG, EMG, and other technologies of conventional medicine. Burr determined that *biologically-based* electricity was no different from that from any other source.

Why has medical science ignored the extraordinary breakthroughs from Professor Harold Burr? Like so many important discoveries, politics, greed and jealousy prevailed—and vital information was swept under the rug. Despite over 40 years of extensive professional publication (*Yale Journal of Biological Medicine*), Dr. Burr's research findings were ignored by the medical community. His work was poorly timed—it came at the time when medicine was certain antibiotics were going to become the "silver bullet"—the cure for all disease. Despite his impressive credentials, Burr's energy-based concepts were not consistent with the biochemical pharmaceutical model of medicine that was exploding on the scene. Although his works can be found in the archives of *Yale Journal of Biology and Medicine*, it is not mentioned in biology textbooks!

How about this for an eerie coincidence:

Dr. Harold Burr conducted research, and lived in Lyme, Connecticut! One of his studies involving elm trees conducted during the 1940s revealed that monitoring changes in electric fields could predict biological activities before they became physically evident. Burr tested L-fields on plant seeds to predict the health of future plants!

Business Trumps Breakthroughs

In 1910, John D. Rockefeller funded the development of a doctrine called the *Flexner Report*. It enabled the AMA to monopolize Western medicine with a focus on pharmaceuticals. The well-executed plan was to eliminate any competition, which included any other treatment approaches. The claim was there were too many doctors and too many medical schools. The *Flexner Report* was positioned as a means of standardizing medical education. It successfully destroyed the development of and usage of natural health care methods—labeling anything other than drugs as unscientific.

With medical schools overhauled as drug-based institutions, electrotherapies (and many other treatments) were banned from medical practice, regardless of effectiveness. The threat of imprisonment was real for those who would continue using them. Essentially, it was the birth of Big Pharma. The AMA has consistently claimed their actions are in the interest of protecting patients. According to Nobel laureate Milton Friedman in his 1961 book, *Capitalism and Freedom* the AMA's attempts to control doctors and their services produced a reduced quality of care and technological advancement. More than fifty years later, little has changed. An academic bias still exists against the bio-energetic model of medicine.

Conventional medicine has been reluctant to pursue bio-energetic research, despite proof that the first sign of diminished health is vibrational or electromagnetic. Frequency damage is stored like computer memory inside your cells. This can accumulate without any outward sign or symptom for years—long before any noticeable chemical or structural damage shows up. With such energetic damage, germs can have more fertile ground to multiply. In other words, it appears that a great deal of disease begins due to electrical interference in our bodies and altered cellular vibrational frequencies, created by a variety of causes.

148

In 1937, Professor Burr determined that abnormal voltage gradients preceded abnormal cellular growth such as cancer. As mentioned, Burr's work has largely been ignored. However, biologists at *Tufts University* recently conducted experiments where they were able to cause frog tadpoles to grow new eyes— by altering electrical voltage on embryonic cells! The researchers concluded that the formation of organs is driven by specific voltages.

(Source: *Transmembrane voltage potential controls embryonic eye patterning in Xenopus* laevis. Pai VP, Aw S, Shomrat T, Lemire JM, Levin M *Development.* 2012 Jan; 139(2):313-23)

The implication is that bio-energetic stimuli interact with genetics to create developments in living systems. This is precisely what Harold Burr was proclaiming so many decades ago. We owe a debt of gratitude to scientists like Harold Burr. He was willing to further medical science at a time when the body was viewed as a machine whose ailments were to be managed chemically with drugs, or mechanically with surgery. You will soon understand how bio-energetic methods could be the key to your recovery from tick-triggered illness.

(Source: Harold Saxton Burr, *Blueprint for immortality; the electric patterns of life.* (1972).

An entire list of Burr's work can be found in the archives of *Yale Journal of Biology and Medicine.* Many academic papers from Dr. Burr can be found at the US National Library of Medicine National Institutes of Health website: http://www.ncbi.nlm.nih.gov

"When one door closes, another opens; but we often look so long and so regretfully upon the closed door that we do not see the one which has opened for us." - Alexander Graham Bell

Chapter 20

Look to the Auricle

An ancient Greek *oracle* refers to a prophet or shrine through which hidden inspired wisdom was believed to be revealed. What a fascinating coincidence it is that the medical term for the outer ear is the *auricle*. Using modern scientific instruments, the auricle provides otherwise hidden information about the human body that other medical means may not reveal. The outer ear functions as a tiny microcosm of living energy that correlates with and connects to the entire body.

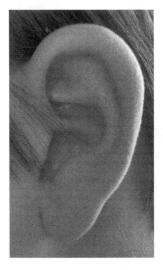

Conventional Western medicine looks to the human ear as only an organ of hearing. It is so much more! The auricle has complicated nerve connections through which constant communication takes place between your ear, brain and the body. There are no direct nerve connections between the ear and every part of the body, but it does indeed have a vast supply of nerve endings connecting it to the brain and spinal cord. It appears that a reflex center in the brain (reticular formation) continuously transmits energy signals to the spinal cord, and then to nerves connecting to the corresponding part of the body.

When there is a disturbance somewhere in your body, a change

150

in the electrical resistance can be detected at pinpoint locations within predictable regions of the skin of the ear. These *temporary* acupuncture points directly correspond to the organs or tissue involved. Stimulating them by various means including acupuncture needles, electrical devices, cold laser, or acupressure pellets can trigger or jump start a natural healing response. This holistic ear-based treatment is called **auricular therapy.** It has been clinically observed to achieve some absolutely stunning results—often after conventional medications and other treatment methods have failed. The *ear* is a key part of the *Bio-energetic Individual Treatment Equation.*

"Up to 1992, I never had a serious illness. It was at that time I discovered I was very allergic to anesthesia. I never fully recovered my strength from an operation. As the years went by my body made many bad changes that could not be cured by western medicine. My immune system failed and became prey to other diseases including Lyme disease. By the time I found Dr. Liebell I was in constant pain and so weak I could not spend a half day awake and out of bed... I was so impressed with his non-invasive bio-energetic testing method and the Auricular Therapy ear acupuncture. Dr. Liebell started me on a weekly pain treatment and a full spectrum of homeopathic remedies... My pain is gone most days and my days of total exhaustion are a thing of the past... It makes me feel so good when people tell me how much better I look now than I did a year ago. I tell them it is all thanks to Dr. Liebell."

- Roberta R., Maryland 2011

Ancient Chinese Secret?

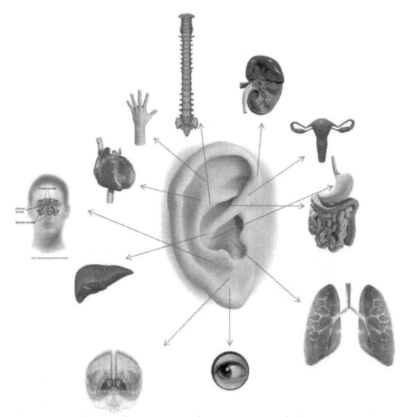

The ear has been documented as an area of therapeutic focus dating back to ancient Egypt, Greece, Rome and Persia. Various sources inaccurately cite auricular therapy to be developed by the Chinese. Auricular therapy is actually a *French* innovation. Historically, Chinese acupuncture involved merely a few points on the ear as part of the comprehensive, full-body meridian energy channel system. In Traditional Chinese medicine (TCM), acupuncture points are very specifically anatomically located at fixed positions on everybody. These are perpetually electrically active—they can always be detected on everybody with instruments.

On the other hand, with auricular therapy there are no exact fixed points; they are constantly changing. They can differ in location on the ear from person to person, within large zones. They exist as electrically detectable acupuncture points if, and only if a problem exists—like the warning light on the dashboard of a car that turns on in case of malfunction.

French Made

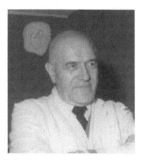

The development of the science of auricular therapy is credited to Paul Nogier, M.D. (1908-1996). He was a conventionally-trained neurologist, who also had an engineering background. He taught at the medical school in Lyon, France. During the 1950s, Dr. Nogier noticed a strange scar on the upper ear of some of his patients. The doctor learned these marks were created by a woman from Marseille named Madame Barrin. Although she was not a doctor, she somehow learned how to intentionally *burn* a certain spot on the outer ear in order to relieve their low back and thigh pain (sciatica). She had no idea why or how it worked. Amazed and fascinated by this unheard of procedure, Dr. Nogier observed it, and performed the same procedure on his own sciatica patients with some success.

With side effects of drugs being a concern, Dr. Nogier sought methods of treatment that worked on a physical and energetic plane, rather than chemical. Thus, the professor studied homeopathic medicine, manual spinal correction, and acupuncture. He reasoned that needling the ear rather than burning it might be a much gentler, less drastic, yet equally effective approach. He was right on the money! Eventually, Dr. Nogier determined that this fantastic sciatica spot was a reflex point that corresponded directly with the fifth lumbar vertebra and its neighboring sacroiliac joint. This is where the sciatic nerve exits the spine, and runs down the leg. Despite the lack of scientific validation, Nogier persisted with detailed investigation of this phenomenon. He keenly hypothesized that if this spot on the ear was effective in treating low back pain, maybe *other* parts of the ear could treat other parts of the body too. Through extensive experimentation, Dr. Nogier systematically mapped out energetic ear reflex projection zones for the entire body.

In a fascinating development, he observed that pattern could be compared to an upside-down human fetus!

The head projects electrical changes to lower ear lobe, the feet at the top of the ear, and the rest of the body in-between. This model was first presented in France in 1957, then spread to Germany, and finally was translated into Chinese. In 1958 the Chinese embraced and adopted this model of acupuncture that was previously unknown to them despite thousands of years of acupuncture practice. They acknowledged Dr. Paul Nogier

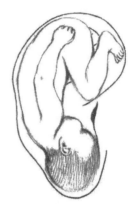

Image: by permission from Soliman's Auricular Therapy Textbook

as the Father of Auricular Therapy. Not satisfied with these initial extraordinary findings, he continued research for decades. Nogier understood that the human body functions through always-changing, and highly dynamic systems. Eventually, he and his research team determined this remarkable inverted fetus presentation to be merely one of *three* possible energy projection patterns that reflected problems in the body!

Every part of the body has three distinct areas or zones for which electrical changes could develop. These are called *auricular energy phases*.

Which zone develops electrical changes depends upon nature of the problem. A sudden or acute condition causes changes in a pinpoint area of one particular zone. A chronic problem results in electrical activity in another zone, quite a distance away. Any physical changes, tissue damage, injury, or degeneration leads to electrically detectable ear acupuncture points in yet another distinct area.

Sorry, Cynical Skeptics... it's Science!

The science of auricular therapy has been well documented, internationally researched, with over 800 papers published in peer-reviewed medical journals. It is not only taught in France, but all of Europe—especially Germany. It is practiced by several thousand European medical doctors. In 1990, Hiroshi Nakajima, the Director General of the *World Health Organization* (WHO) praised Dr. Paul Nogier, and encouraged medical doctors to use auricular therapy. Despite its success, most North American doctors are unfamiliar with it. Auricular therapy has proven to bring pain relief and support healing, in many cases, after all other medical interventions have failed.

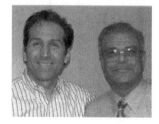

Around 1995, Nogier's authentic work was brought to America, brilliantly re-vitalized, refined, and furthered by anesthesiologist, medical acupuncturist and homeopathy expert, **Nader Soliman, M.D.** I am proud and privileged to have been personally trained by him. Gleaning from Dr. Soliman's experience, I have been thrilled to serve Americans by carrying on the noble work of Dr. Paul Nogier.

The reticular formation of the brain collects information from the entire body, and sends it to the ear. This is why the outer ear (the auricle) reflects everything going on in the body, and what the brain is trying to do to deal with it. The ear serves as a hologram decoder! For more details about the scientific validity of auricular therapy, explore the section dedicated to it at my ear-based website:

http://www.liebellclinic.com/auricular-therapy-ear-acupuncture-research.html

Soldiers' Attention!

Auricular therapy was successfully implemented into the *United States Armed Forces* thanks to recently retired Air Force Colonel Richard C. Niemtzow, M.D., Ph.D., M.P.H. He is a radiation oncologist, who became the first full-time physician acupuncturist for the U.S. Armed Forces. Dr. Niemtzow teaches military physicians an auricular technique called *"Battlefield Acupuncture."* He established an extremely popular clinic at *Andrews Air Force Base*, where he serves personnel from *Andrews*, the *Pentagon, White House, National Naval Medical Center*, and *Walter Reed Army Medical Center.* Dr. Niemtzow is currently (2015) Consultant for Alternative Medicine for the *United States Air Force Surgeon General.* He also represents the *Department of Defense* at the *National Institutes of Health, National Center for Complementary and Alternative Medicine Advisory Council.*

What in the world does your *ear* have to do with overcoming chronic tick-triggered illness? The answer is everything! The auricular therapy component just scratches the surface. In the upcoming chapters, you will learn how the auricle gives us the answers.

"The electro-dynamic fields which control the human organism are signposts to the most promising trail that future explorers can follow" – Dr. Harold Saxton Burr, (1889-1973) *Professor Emeritus of Anatomy, Yale University Medical School*

Chapter 21

An Earful of Wisdom

How the Ear is Used to Determine Treatment Needs... and Why it Does NOT Matter Whether or Not You Have Been "Officially" Diagnosed With Lyme Disease

You feel just plain lousy. You've been submitted to every kind of physical examination and test your doctors can administer. You've given blood and urine. You've had x-rays, MRI, CT-scans, nerve tests... but everything comes up negative. There is no *visible or measurable damage.* Lyme disease blood tests may come up negative—even if you *know* you were bitten by a tick... even if you've had an expanding red rash (bull's eye or similar). The Western Blot Lyme test has a strict requirement for an official positive. If you don't meet the full requirement, Lyme disease is ruled out and you are given a clean bill of health. This "standard" medical test can leave you in the lurch—scratching your head in disbelief, as your mysterious misery persists. In other words, you've got to be *visibly* sick enough to be considered sick! Next you're hearing about a trip to the psychiatrist.

Mainstream medicine functions primarily when there is visible damage, or observable and measurable phenomena using conventional medical devices. In order to receive an official medical diagnosis, one must exhibit such findings, however, it is often the case that these present themselves only when substantial damage has taken place. Catching illness before it takes *physical* form is still not within the realm of conventional medicine. It *could* be, as Dr. Harold Burr proclaimed decades ago. In the field of energy medicine, we understand that we can gain further insight into human health by observing the subtle electromagnetic energies of the body, when chemical and physical medical evaluation comes up empty.

Selective Attention in Medicine

Doctors and researchers can have selective attention. By this I mean they tend to only see what they are expecting to, or want to see, but little else. Nobel prize-winning researchers, Drs. Daniel Simons and Christopher Chabris refer to this as *perceptual blindness*—the failure to notice something significant and obvious. To illustrate this point, Simons and Chabris conducted one of the best-known experiments in psychology (1999). Viewers are asked to watch a very short video of six people passing around basketballs. Three of them are wearing white shirts, and the other three black shits. The instructions are to watch the video and count to yourself how many times the white-shirted people pass the basketball. Twenty-three seconds into the video, a *gorilla* walks in between the ball players, stops and beats its chest and walks off—for a total of nine seconds spent prominently on screen. Yet, half the people who watch this video do not notice the gorilla, as if it were invisible. Try it out with other people:

https://www.youtube.com/watch?v=vJG698U2Mvo

Chabris and Simon say this experiment reveals that we miss a lot of what goes on around us, and that we are unaware that we do so. Why have I referenced this ingenious experiment? "Invisible gorillas" are rampantly lurking about in our bodies. However, they are rarely seen, because doctors are too busy looking for *other* things. They expect to find what conventional evaluation permits, and thus they may not pursue valuable information that could be ferreted out by other means. Many doctors are guilty of overlooking "invisible gorillas." Simon and Chabris assert that experts are actually *more* prone to inattentional blindness than beginners. Experts typically have specific expectations based upon experience, so they "know" what to expect to find in certain situations. They become blind to the unexpected, even if it is staring them right in the face. This brings us to the subject of this chapter. There must be a way to help people--that doesn't depend on the faulty blood tests, and a politically corrupt and questionable system that is obsessed with antibiotics, and naming people with disease syndromes. And there IS.

At the heart of the BITE is a unique evaluation method, called **Auricular Bio-energetic Testing** (ABT). It is a sophisticated, complex, and fascinating way of using electromagnetic signals of the body to give health information, and to predict the effectiveness of various treatments for each individual. Many decades ago, Dr. Harold Burr proved that our bodies project a living electromagnetic field (L-field or bio-energetic field). He had hoped that doctors would someday be able to utilize electrical instruments to measure these fields. To this day, no such machines are used medically. However, Dr. Paul Nogier developed a method for measuring fluctuations of the human electric field *without* a machine! During the late 1960s, prompted by his acupuncture studies, Nogier began taking his patients' pulse at the wrist, while examining their ears. He noticed a stronger or fuller pulse could be felt for a few seconds when he touched certain areas of the ear. Nogier determined that this reflex of the cardiovascular and nervous systems happens all the time upon stress, and that it could be intentionally elicited for examination purposes.

Dr. Paul Nogier lived during a time of tremendous scientific advancement, at the crossroads between cultures. Although he had been trained in conventional medicine, he also understood the Chinese concepts that living things are governed by energy. This enabled him to discover the Nogier pulse reflex. The art of evaluating cardiovascular function for various medical purposes has a rich history. For over 3,000 years, the Chinese made use of monitoring pulses to develop acupuncture. However, the Chinese were not aware of electromagnetic waves. Neither Western medicine nor traditional Chinese medicine had known of Nogier's application of this pulse reflex. It is a very subtle, normal, and predictable muscle contraction that can be felt in the arteries. He incorporated it into the auricular therapy system he introduced a decade earlier. He originally called this advancement auricular *medicine*.

Through extensive research and experimentation with this pulse reflex, Nogier discovered that under non-stressful and healthy circumstances, our ears project a normal electromagnetic field that extends outwards less than ½ an inch. But in sickness or stress, this electromagnetic field can expand up to several feet. Through his experiments, Nogier determined that we can see the bio-energetic field distance by intentionally trigger the pulse reflex. He used very specific frequencies of Kodak-Wratten color light filters. Gliding the filter towards the ear triggers the Nogier's pulse reflex upon contact with the patient's bio-electric field. Thus, we can observe how far away it is from the ear when the pulse feels fuller. Picture a balloon inflating slightly. That is what is felt by the doctor in the artery at the wrist. It is a very delicate procedure, which requires very well-trained and experienced hands, and a fine sense of touch to consistently and reliably detect the Nogier reflex.

Doctors listen to the heartbeat through a stethoscope. Blood pressure, heart rate, and other functions can be measured through various technologies. At this point in time, interest in the application of the Nogier reflex is still in its infancy, even though he developed it decades ago. Dr. Paul Nogier was decorated for his contributions to medicine by the French government.

To avoid confusion, I refer to auricular medicine as **Auricular Bio-energetic Testing** (ABT). Some practitioners who perform auricular *therapy* (ear acupuncture) refer to their services as auricular medicine. Perhaps they do so because medicine sounds more impressive than therapy, or they simply do not know the difference. Although popular and successful in Europe, a handful of American doctors correctly utilize Nogier's advanced techniques. ABT was further developed in the U.S. by anesthesiologist, medical acupuncturist, and homeopath, Nader Soliman, M.D.

There are four main principles involved in Auricular Bio-energetic Testing:

1. Bio-Electric Fields
2. Auricular Therapy Ear Acupuncture Micro-System
3. The Nogier Pulse Reflex – a Cardiovascular Response
4. Physics Principles of Resonance and Frequencies

In previous chapters, you have already learned about bio-electric fields and auricular therapy. Now that you have been introduced to the Nogier pulse reflex, here is the final component of Auricular Bio-energetic Testing:

Resonance Phenomenon

Physicists know that matter and energy waves vibrate at a specific frequency per unit of time. In the 1600s, Galileo discovered the principle of **resonance.** It is widely observed in nature, and it is extensively utilized in human technology.

Resonance is the mechanism by which virtually all vibrations are generated. Many sounds we hear, such as when hard objects of metal, glass, or wood are struck, are caused by brief resonant vibrations in the object. Light and electromagnetic fields are produced by resonance on an atomic level.

Resonance occurs when energy is transferred between two or more sources of that vibrate at the same frequency. It is an energetic connection or matching of frequencies. Every object has a resonant frequency. This means that if you hit, pluck or heat it—it will vibrate at a specific rate. This is the case with musical instruments, such as a drum, a guitar string or a xylophone. Each distinct musical note is the result of a vibrational frequency. If two different objects naturally vibrate at a certain frequency, they can become energetically connected… even without touching. This can be easily demonstrated with tuning forks of the same frequency. Or think of an opera singer who can break a wine glass by singing a certain note. She is energetically connecting with the exact frequency of the glass, causing its atoms to vibrate so violently that the glass shatters. Another example of resonance in action is the electronic keypad that unlocks the door of your car. It emits a specific frequency that resonates only with your vehicle to let you in.

Dr. Nogier found that with Auricular Bio-energetic Testing, the principle of resonance could be utilized to gain insight to our health. Energetic clues that an organ is stressed, injured, or diseased can be found through resonance matching. This is accomplished using professionally prepared liquid samples containing the energetic imprints of the frequencies of toxins, microbes, diseased tissues, organs, hormones, and chemicals. No live microbes or biological tissues are used. Since all substances have a specific frequency, we can briefly stress the body with a test sample to see if a resonance or a vibrational match exists. If a stressed organ, microbe, or a substance exists

162

in your body, and we connect an additional energetic stimulus of more of the same frequency—your bio-energetic field will project farther away from your ears.

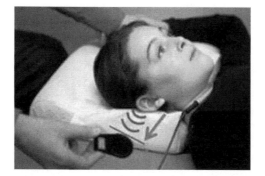

The samples are placed on metal plates, which are connected to you by wires and electrode bars. One bar is held in your hand, and the other is placed on your neck or belly. Although there is no machinery involved, this creates a living electromagnetic circuit—perfect for energetic testing. Throughout the exam, dozens of samples are added and subtracted from the plates, and we observe how they affect the bio-electric field distance. It is akin to asking the nervous system questions… and getting answers that cannot be obtained through physical tests.

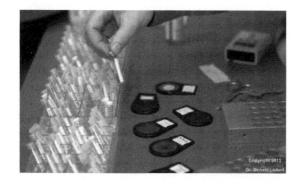

Case Example: A 47-year-old woman suffered for 6 years from headaches, fatigue, dizziness, and various body pains. All physical tests, X-rays, MRI, CT Scans and blood test were negative. She had been given various medications to treat the symptoms, which at best provide temporary relief. She was given the diagnoses of Fibromyalgia and Migraines. Unhappy with diagnosis without evidence, and treatment that never address the cause of her symptoms, she sought out the BITE. A thorough case history led me to suspect some possible causes. We measured her baseline electric field distance at a quite abnormal 10 inches (normal is less than half an inch). Adding a resonance sample of the frequencies of brain tissue to the test plate connected to her hand caused her electric field expanded to nearly 2 feet off her ear!

The next step was to see what toxins or microbes might be stressing her brain. A frequency resonance sample of *Borrelia*— the bacteria of Lyme disease was added to the test plate connected by wire to the skin of her neck. Re-testing her bio-electric field revealed a reduction to less than one inch. This was an energetic suggestion—an inference that the cause of her head-related symptoms was Lyme disease. To further establish this, the *Borrelia* sample was switched to the plate connected to the patient's hand, along with the brain sample. Her bio-electric field projected nearly 3 feet from her ear.

Finally, a sample of a bio-energetic supplement product was added to the same plate. The added energetic frequencies of the proposed treatment brought her electric field to less than one inch. This question and answer-like approach was used for this and other areas of her body, and various samples of possible causative agents. This provided direction for determining ear acupuncture treatment and a customized homeopathic protocol for her. She had given conventional medications and diagnosis ample opportunity to help her, with no improvement. In under six months, using the homeopathic and acupuncture protocol, she was headache and dizziness free, with a marked decrease in body pains.

Bi-Digital O-Ring Test (BDORT)

Bi-Digital O-Ring Test (BDORT) is another valuable bio-energetic method. It is a patented diagnostic method which was invented, developed, and patented by world-renowned oncologist, cardiologist, acupuncturist, medical school professor and research scientist, 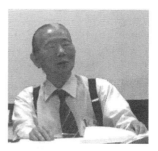 Yoshiaki Omura, MD. His remarkable background in both Western and Eastern medicine, as well as physics, and electronics has given him remarkable scientific qualifications (http://bdort.org/about-omura.html).

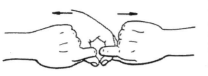 BDORT is performed by the patient forming an O-shaped ring with the thumb and one other finger. The testing doctor uses a structured series of tests where he/she tries to pull apart the patient's O-ring with fingers in the same orientation. This is performed while the patient is in contact with (or connected by wire to) whatever sample is being used for testing. These may include supplements, laboratory-prepared microscope slides of organs and tissues, resonance samples (technological facsimiles of substances) or virtually any other material.

Like Auricular Bio-energetic Testing (ABT), BDORT is a test of interaction of the electromagnetic field of the internal organs and whatever sample is being utilized. With this approach, feedback comes in the form of temporary changes in muscular resistance (weakening of O-ring of the patient). BDORT is a reproducible, non-invasive, and inexpensive objective medical testing method. Like standard laboratory medical tests, BDORT is a measuring technique. It is used to evaluate if any stimulus

165

results in either a temporary increase or decrease in finger muscle strength. This provides insights to what is going on in the body. BDORT is a bio-energetic evaluation method that gives us valuable clues without exposing patients to radiation, imaging dyes and other hazardous diagnostic testing factors. I have found patients to be fascinated by this non-invasive, rapid, safe, and effective means of determining the nature of health problems, and subsequent treatment.

How Does BDORT Work?

Using BDORT, the practitioner can test whether a substance (or other stimulus) makes the body weaker or stronger (or neutral effect). This is done by making muscle strength comparisons in response to adding or subtracting different stimuli, such as samples of supplements, foods, chemicals, herbs, homeopathic remedies. A licensed medical doctor can use BDORT to test prescription medications.

All substances have specific electromagnetic properties, which are good, bad, or neutral in their effect on one's body. If a harmful substance is held by the patient, it creates a temporary muscle weakness, due to a brain response. By contrast, beneficial substances and other stimuli produce strengthening. With both ABT and BDORT, we are using the phenomenon of physics known as **resonance** to determine likely effectiveness and optimal dosages of supplements, as well as compatibility of them with other substances.

BDORT is a test of interaction of the electromagnetic field of the internal organs and whatever sample is being utilized. Feedback comes in the form of temporary changes in muscular resistance (either strengthening or weakening of O-ring of the patient). With BDORT, we are observing physiological response upon introducing various stimuli to the body—to see if and how they resonate with the body. If a substance that is harmful

166

to a person is held, the O-ring weakens. By contrast, holding something *beneficial* produces immediate strengthening. This can be a supportive food, supplement, homeopathic remedy, medicine, touching an acupuncture point, etc. The reason bio-energetic evaluations such as BDORT and ABT work is that we are electromagnetic beings. The fundamental nature of life is bio-energetic! It is fantastic to be able to investigate and determine problems in the body, non-invasively. BDORT is a method of comparative measurement. Testing muscle strength has long been a universally-accepted conventional medical method of determining neurological integrity and related problems.

The foundation for using comparative muscle response is the work of chiropractor, Dr. George Goodhart. In 1964, he observed that muscles go weak in response to harmful stimuli, but strengthen from beneficial stimuli. He called it Applied Kinesiology. However, because it was a technology-free approach (combined with the American Medical Association's unethical bias towards chiropractors), it has been poorly accepted. In 1977, Dr. Omura introduced BDORT. It is a thoroughly researched, developed, documented, and advanced system of muscle testing. It is performed by following a specific and strict set of rules. Dr. Omura spent over seven years of evaluation before the U.S. Patent Office granted him approval for BDORT (1993). According to Dr. Omura, it was almost rejected because his method seemed too unbelievable to be true. Despite what skeptics and critics have stated, BDORT was never rejected; the patent office merely was interested in more clinical evidence, which Dr. Omura supplied successfully, under the scrutiny of a large panel of medical investigators. To the best of my knowledge, BDORT is the only patented and proven bio-energetic testing method. I think it is quite impressive to be awarded a patent for the use of the human body as a medical diagnostic tool.

With both ABT and BDORT, we can get important information about the body without drawing blood, needle biopsies, x-rays, CT scans (CT scans are equivalent to the radiation of 100-500 x-rays!). BDORT has been accepted in Japanese medicine, and it works well in conjunction with both eastern and western medical practices. Even with Dr. Omura's impressive conventional medical credentials, published research, and U.S. patent; BDORT is not taken seriously.

I take it VERY seriously!

Dr. Omura has researched and developed BDORT as a non-invasive method of detecting various cancers, infections, and biochemical changes in the body. He uses it as part of his new method of evaluating electrocardiograms (ECG). BDORT often indicates abnormality in the heart, even though these ECGs are considered within normal limits according to conventional diagnosis standards. **Dr. Omura has concluded that Lyme disease bacterial infection is one of the major causes of atrial fibrillation, a common heart condition.** In 1986 (using BDORT), Dr. Omura discovered that the *Helicobacter pylori* bacteria was involved with stomach ulcers and cancer. This was way before Australian scientists were awarded the 2005 Nobel Prize for the *same* discovery!

BDORT has indeed been studied extensively, and much of its mechanism is scientifically understood and verified. Despite this, it has not received mainstream attention (and it likely will not). Mainstream medicine does not appear to be fond of inexpensive diagnostic methods that do not require high-tech devices. Most standard medical tests are based upon chemical reactions and measurements. The focus of BDORT is the phenomenon of electromagnetic resonance, which is the underlying force of chemical reactions. One can cogently argue that such bio-energetic investigation is *more* sophisticated than the chemical and structural abnormality-based approach to diagnosis. Medical doctors, who take the opportunity to use BDORT, can use it as an effective tool for choosing prescription medications and their dosages. This is a magnificent application! Instead of merely guessing what drug might be effective, Dr. Omura uses his fast and safe method to see what medication may be better suited or not for a patient. I am a doctor of chiropractic (DC) and am also licensed by the Virginia Board of Medicine in acupuncture. I do not prescribe medications, nor do I advise patients regarding their usage. Therefore, I only use BDORT applications for drug-free treatments (bio-energetic supplements, foods, other non-pharmaceutical substances, homeopathic remedies, acupuncture, vitamins and minerals, etc.).

I encourage you to watch the remarkable 45-minute documentary on the BDORT produced by Tokai Television (Nogoya City, Japan) in 1992. It is Japan's equivalent to NOVA, which we see on American public television. The English dubbing is quite good. It was made at a medical school, dental school, and major Japanese hospital. You will see how the doctors use BDORT to pinpoint a 5mm stomach cancer in a woman, in only 30 minutes. Then, it is confirmed with follow-up independent diagnosis using conventional laboratory tests including: contrast x-ray, and fiber-optic stomach scoping with a chemical dye, and biopsy. Identical results were obtained by BDORT and these extremely expensive tests!

http://bdort.org/videos.html

One might hope that such a method would transform modern medicine. This might be the case if popularizing it would not have devastating financial impact on the medical industry. Clearly, the masses are trusting contemporary conventional medical methods over anything else. It is considered appropriate to perform exorbitantly expensive, risky, and invasive diagnostics tests first, and prescribe chemical medicines. The

169

public is accustomed to this, and has also been well-trained to be fearful of anything else as a consideration. Medical research focuses mostly on discoveries that lead to expensive solutions. Everybody knows this is true. How long has the public been promised cures for cancer? How many billions of dollars will continue to be spent? The FDA is the rule of law that says essentially one must never claim to cure anything (and I do not).

Conventional treatment of chronic pain and illness is big business. I am proud to make it a very *small* business! Meeting people whose lives have been saved by Dr. Omura is life changing. You will learn in Chapter 29 how I learned from Dr. Omura how to further help people by determining their optimal dosage of vitamin D supplementation (a critical factor for countless health problems). It is quite inspirational to see an 84-year-old man continue to conduct research, and fly around the world to help people and further medicine.

Dr. Yoshiaki Omura is likely the most capable person on the planet for early detection of cancer, and determining what promotes improvement (and worsening) Dr. Omura's research and recommendations do not involve promotion or sales of anything; they serve to enable people to have a fighting chance to live and get healthier. He does not have a blog, a marketing newsletter, an Omura product line, nor does he sell diagnostic equipment. Helping seriously ill people, very inexpensively, and without the use of fancy technology is not taken seriously by mainstream medicine, regardless of outcome. It is this aspect that especially attracted me to study the methods of Dr. Yoshiaki Omura. If Dr. Omura talks; I'm listening!

Many patients who seek my support for the fight against tick-triggered illness, have been told by previous physicians that their diagnostic tests are normal—that nothing wrong can be found. Yet their symptoms persist. There must be causes despite a lack of evidence from blood tests, x-rays, and MRI and other diagnostic technologies. This is when bio-energetic testing shines. Mainstream medical governing bodies do not currently acknowledge these energetic observations as diagnostic proof of any medical condition, nor do I represent them as such. Nevertheless, they have been the means by which patients have been guided towards recovery. What is always fascinating to patients is when ABT and BDORT observations concur with the findings of *physical and laboratory* tests. In some cases, bio-energetic findings (in absence of symptoms or tissue damage of a developing underlying condition) will lead us to pursue conventional medical diagnostic testing, which might not be otherwise considered. This can provide important insights to the best treatments possible from both conventional and holistic medicine. This is precisely what Dr. Harold Burr (mentioned in Chapter 19) likely envisioned.

The first major step towards getting better is to accept that your *real* condition is a dysfunctional immune system—not Lyme disease. That is the fundamental principle of the *Bio-energetic Individual Treatment Equation.*© The goal of bio-energetic testing is to utilize the subtle electromagnetic energy fields of the body to obtain useful feedback for helping patients. We seek to discover weakness and imbalances, and in turn, determine effective means to correct them—before they lead to further chemical and structural damage.

Both Auricular Bio-energetic Testing (ABT) and Bi-Digital O-Ring Testing (BDORT) are *clinical examination methods*, not machines or diagnostic technologies. Applying the principles of either the Nogier pulse reflex or O-ring muscle testing are additional medical approaches to deciphering the mysteries of the human body. The Nogier pulse ABT method is based on touch (palpation) of the radial pulse at the wrist. Mastering the nuances and the touch sensitivity and skills required for ABT has been a daunting, but rewarding task of many years. It could be compared to a blind person developing the skills to read

171

Braille. There has yet to be developed a scientific instrument capable of competing with touch sensitivity and perception of the practitioner. If such would be created, it might change the whole face of medicine. Perhaps that is why it has not been done! We hope that someday, financing research to develop such technology will become a priority. Several years ago, I proposed such a project to the health sciences department of a major Virginia state university. They claimed to be interested in research involving bio-electric therapies, but passed on the opportunity.

I am humbled by the genius of Dr. Nogier. And I am forever grateful and proud to be trained in Auricular Bio-energetic Testing by Nader Soliman, M.D. Dr. Soliman has helped me to carry on the work of Dr. Paul Nogier—to serve the health needs of those who have lost hope. Without it, my wife would still have Tick-triggered illness. We hope to see more doctors demonstrate the open-mindedness to explore human health care methods outside the realm of conventional drug and surgical practices. Dr. Paul Nogier was ahead of his time. I am very proud to carry on his work, using the methods that have meant the world to my family, and I'm proud to say, to the wonderful people who have given me the opportunity to help them naturally recover from chronic tick-triggered illness. ABT is not yet a medically-accepted means to diagnose any medical conditions, including Lyme disease. We refer to observations made with both ABT and BDORT as **energetic suggestions** or inferences. These methods provide the doctor with fantastic clues for making treatment decisions. Combined with medical history and consultation, they are magnificent means by which each individual's wellness-promoting protocol (including auricular therapy/ear acupuncture) can be determined. I am humbled by the genius of Dr. Paul Nogier. If he were living today, I'd pay to listen to him mumble in his sleep!

172

"The day science begins to study non-physical phenomena, it will make more progress in one decade than in all the previous centuries of its existence." — Nikola Tesla

Chapter 22

Clearing Energetic Blockages of the Brain: The First Step Towards Recovery

Many factors may disrupt the flow of energy, which can have far-reaching consequences to our health. Energetic blockages are obstacles to the normal energy flow throughout the body. Eastern medicine acknowledges that health depends upon energetic balance and stability of the body-mind-spirit axis.

In traditional Chinese medicine (TCM), symptoms of blockages are described as disruptions to the flow of Qi (living energy of the body) through the well-established acupuncture meridian channels. They are detected and treated by various means, depending on the techniques and approach of the practitioner. Scars are a large focus for blockages in TCM. Detecting and eliminating energetic blockages is one of the cornerstones of acupuncture, regardless of discipline or technique. It is no surprise that most Western medicine practitioners have historically rejected the concept. This is, fortunately, of no consequence, since acupuncture patients have thrived for thousands of years.

Modern research and technology is now scientifically verifying this principle that has been understood for thousands of years by many cultures. Auricular therapy and Auricular Bio-energetic Testing (ABT) are at the forefront of the scientific energy medicine revolution. When one undergoes ABT, the first step for all patients is to check for energetic blockages, and treat them accordingly using Neuro-electric Therapy (an electrical frequency acupuncture treatment) and/or specialized ear acupuncture needles.

Energetic blockages can stall or prevent your body from doing the job that it would otherwise be capable of, which may result in chronic pain and illness. The beauty of clearing energetic blockages with acupuncture techniques is that a person may start to naturally improve with little or any further medical intervention. Sometimes in my practice, I do a procedure that seems so easy, quick, painless, and simple that it seems like it shouldn't be able to have any effect. Yet, one needle (and/or electrical) treatment to the right area will often unleash a healing response that can be explained by nothing else—because no prior treatment efforts were successful. It's like knowing where a light switch is to illuminate a dark room, and simply turning it on.

It is not difficult to understand the concept of a mechanical or physical blockage, such as a dam blocking the flow of water in a river. A clogged artery obviously can be a deadly blockage. A less obvious type of blockage can exist due to mechanically malfunctioning functioning joints. This can result in inflammation that in turn, blocks normal nerve function. This is an energetic blockage caused by mechanical problem. It is not a coincidence that so many traditional Chinese acupuncture points exist near joints.

The first part of evaluation when applying the *Bio-energetic Individual Therapy Equation* is detecting and clearing energetic blockages—particularly those that correlate with brain structures. Others may be detected in various other structures, including certain joints and nerves. These are blockages discovered by Dr. Paul Nogier of France

174

by means of Auricular Bio-energetic Testing, which he developed. They were not known to traditional Chinese medicine. Additional blockages have been discovered by Dr. Nader Soliman, who has furthered and modernized Nogier's work. Such blockages are not physical problems, such as a growth, tumor, or calcification that could be seen on x-ray, MRI, or CT-scan. The field of bio-energetic medicine concerns itself with electromagnetic changes in the body.

The Corpus Callosum

The corpus callosum is a wide, thick bundle of nerve fibers in the brain. It is composed of approximately 250 million nerve fibers. We have one brain, but it is divided into two sides or hemispheres by the corpus callosum. It is the information superhighway between the left and right sides (hemispheres) of the brain. It is the pathway of transfer for information pertaining to your senses, movement, and thinking from the two sides of the brain. It is also involved in eye movement, balance, and your sense of touch.

The LEFT hemisphere of the brain is generally associated with math, logic, and language. The RIGHT hemisphere's functions are spatial ability, visual imagery, music, and face recognition. Keep in mind that the right and left brain are connected. Sharing information between the left and right hemispheres of the brain is the function of the corpus callosum. The right side of your brain controls the muscles and most sensory information of the left side of your body. The left brain controls the same functions on the right. This is why damage to one side of the brain impairs the opposite side of the body.

Normal corpus callosum function is critical to recovery from various health problems. There are many named conditions in conventional medical diagnosis that can be associated with communications problem with the corpus callosum, such as:

175

attention deficit disorder, dyslexia, stuttering, difficulty with following directions or making choices (brain fog?), balance problems, emotional fragility, and others. A great deal of the scientific knowledge regarding the hemispheres of the brain comes from surgery, where the right and left sides are intentionally split. However, in conventional medicine, unless there is visible structural damage, or measurable chemical changes—a diagnosis of corpus callosum malfunction is unlikely to be made, and certainly no treatment would be rendered.

If there is a problem with the corpus callosum, electrical changes become detectable on the ear. There will be one or more pinpoint spots found somewhere within three potential large areas. There is no standard corpus callosum acupuncture point on the ear. A high percentage of victims of tick-triggered illness have blockage of the corpus callosum. Like a faulty electric circuit, this can result in altered communication between the left and right hemispheres of the brain. I have seen in many cases where merely treating ear points correlated with the corpus callosum have broken the cycle of pain or other bodily dysfunction.

Pineal Gland

Energetic blockage to the pineal gland of the brain is another common and critical consideration. The pineal gland is a brain structure that has great importance to many bodily functions. It is discussed in detail in the chapter on sleep, with emphasis on the substances melatonin and serotonin. We commonly find energetic blockages to the pineal gland in cases of chronic tick-triggered illness. Like other energetic blockages of brain structures, the pineal gland cannot be directly affected by meridian-based traditional acupuncture. Approximately 80% of patients reporting for the effects of tick-triggered illness demonstrate pineal problems.

176

The R-Zone: The Reactional Brain

There is potential brain blockage that can occur at several regions that overlap. They were designated by Dr. Paul Nogier and his fellow researcher, Dr. Rene Bourdiol as the "R" Zone. It has also been referred to as the psycho-analytical point. Blockage to the "R" zone can drastically impair healing. I have found many patients, who believed all of their symptoms were caused by Lyme disease to have "R" zone energetic blockages. Once cleared, improvements in cognitive function can be rapid and lasting. It is not unusual for a patient who has received auricular therapy at this area to notice a change in recollection of dreams—often associated with past trauma. This appears to enable the release of such trauma. This is of course, significant for those suffering PTSD.

The Amygdala

The amygdala is a brain structure that plays a major role in a wide variety of human emotions and memory. Problems with the amygdala may be associated with conditions such as depression, anxiety, phobias, post-traumatic stress disorder, and even autism. This energetic blockage, along with those involving the cingulate gyrus, and hippocampus were recently discovered by Nader Soliman, M.D. I have found amygdala blockage to exist in a many of my patients. Performing auricular therapy has produced great patient satisfaction.

Cingulate Gyrus

This part of the brain is involved with processing life situations and adapting to them. What one sees, and how one responds physically and emotionally are in part, processed by the cingulate gyrus. Flexibility in dealing with different situations is one of its functions. How one behaves in school or work versus horsing around privately with friends is an example. It is thought that those who exhibit road rage may have a cingulate gyrus problem.

Hippocampus

The hippocampus plays a major role in memory retention. It is involved with converting recent memories into long-term memory. The hippocampus also has functions regarding spatial relationships.

"The Key to the House"

It is thought that energetic blockages can be the result of physical or emotion trauma, heavy metal toxicity, chemicals, and of perhaps greatest significance, chronic infection. There is no doubt that further scientific investigation into the blockage phenomenon would produce stunning revelations. Clinical results certainly demonstrate the urgency for addressing them. Energetic blockages interfere with optimum body function. Think of electric circuitry that is flawed. Before any type of further treatment is rendered, energetic blockages must be cleared. Otherwise, any subsequent treatment—no matter how magnificent, may be doomed to failure.

Picture a big house that is in disrepair and dirty on the inside. A cleaning crew, carpenters, plumbers, electricians, and interior decorators stand ready outside to clean, repair, and renovate the place. But there's one major problem: the door is locked, and nobody's got the key! I compare clearing energetic blockages through auricular therapy to unlocking the door to the body—to enable repairs and renovations and the cleanup job to take place (natural and normal detoxification aided by bio-energetic supplement). The tiny acupuncture needles and/or the neuro-electric stimulation serve as the "key."

For Practitioners Only:

Chiropractors, medical doctors, osteopathic physicians, and acupuncturists… the first step in becoming trained to provide extraordinary care through applying the *Bio-energetic Individual Treatment Equation* (BITE) is to purchase **Soliman's Auricular Therapy Textbook.** This book will serve as an incredible resource for effective ear acupuncture for which patients will

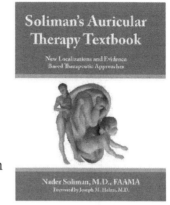

benefit beyond your wildest expectations. No other educational resource will better provide you with the magnificent work of Dr. Paul Nogier and other early pioneers, as well as the knowledge of many outstanding teachers and clinicians, and the experience of today's world authority on auricular therapy, Nader Soliman, M.D.

Then one must attend his instructional seminars at his office in Rockville, Maryland: www.alternativemedicinecenter.info. You will receive training in auricular therapy, auricular bio-energetic testing, and bio-energetic supplementation.

Once technical medical skills are developed, the Liebell Clinic in Virginia Beach provides training in the office procedures necessary to correctly implement the BITE, including: website development and other Internet technology, licensing and usage of educational tools, audio-visual presentations, patient management, and working with the news media: www.liebellclinic.com

"In every culture and in every medical tradition before ours, healing was accomplished by moving energy." - Dr. Albert Szent-Gyorgyi, Nobel laureate in Medicine — *"Introduction to a submolecular biology"*

Chapter 23

Patient-Centered Holistic Wellness

I refer to my patients as victims of tick-triggered illness. People seek my care for the effects of Lyme disease, however I do not diagnose anybody with Lyme disease, chronic Lyme disease, post-treatment Lyme disease syndrome (PTLDS), or any other related label. Providing wellness support for those afflicted by its apparent effects does not constitute medical diagnosis at all. It is no more a treatment for infectious disease than adopting a specific diet or exercise regimen for general health improvement. Treatment of Lyme disease is performed by medical doctors who prescribe antibiotics for medically-proven active *Borrelia* infection. Proving whether or not a person has Lyme disease or many *other* infectious diseases is problematic, at best. Controversy and debate over the existence of chronic Lyme disease has no relevance to my wellness support program. Any person who has experienced a decline in health, and is seeking holistic and natural support may receive it. It does not matter how many (if any) positive bands show up on a Western Blot blood test, or whether or not a bull's eye rash has ever been witnessed.

Various Lyme disease protocols exist named after their respective developers. I respectfully do not mention names, nor is my intention to pass judgment or condemn anybody. In my opinion, doctors ought to leave their egos at the door because the *patient* must always be the center of attention. Forgiving the obvious cliché, patients should be the ones in the limelight. I prefer a less narcissistic description of the services I provide, which is why it is called the *Bio-energetic Individual Treatment Equation.*© It is critical to resist the allure of one-size-fits-all treatment protocols. The goal is to improve your impaired *physiology* rather than try to kill Lyme bacteria. I have reinforced throughout this book that is but one mere pathogen that may be an agent of disease. Generic protocols are NOT holistic, nor do they constitute treating patients as an individual. Lyme disease is the illness caused by the bacterial infection of *Borrelia burgdorferi.* But is this the true condition for which each individual suffers? No. Every person's body expresses different consequences as a result of multiple causes, one of which may be Lyme infection. We must never implement a standardized protocol because human beings are not standardized. We must figure out each patient's specific protocol or treatment regimen.

Human immune systems have been conquering infections for as long as people have roamed the earth. If you can grasp the simple concept that your body can indeed overcome tick-borne infection (and its lingering effects) *itself*—without chemical intervention, you have taken the first step towards recovery and rehabilitation. The task is to support the body's natural inborn ability to overcome multiple causes of pain and illness. Bio-energetic testing is our GPS. It helps navigate us towards effective wellness supporting treatments. This begins with any necessary auricular therapy—particularly clearing energetic blockages. Auricular therapy serves as the "ignition switch." Once accomplished, the stage is set for the body to become mobilized back into action, even if many years of pain and deterioration have been suffered. This is accomplished with bio-energetic wellness supplementation, which serves as our fuel. This ultimate part of the BITE is extremely safe, ridiculously easy-to-do, affordable, and effective. It is free of side effects, drug interactions, and is not dependent upon any medical diagnosis or questionable laboratory tests. It has been my patients' "secret weapon" for natural health recovery.

"Those who merely study and treat the effects of disease are like those who imagine that they can drive away the winter by brushing the snow off the door…It is not the snow that causes winter, but the winter that causes the snow." - Paracelsus (1493-1542)

Chapter 24

Homeopathic Principles to the Rescue!

Although homeopathy has been documented as the second most used health care approach in the world, much confusion exists about it. Much like conventional pharmaceutical medicine, homeopathy has a wide variety of applications, approaches, and forms of usage.

Here are some quick facts, for starters:

- Homeopathic medicine has been a fixture in health care around the world for over 200 years. In the early 1900s, there were nearly two dozen American medical schools teaching homeopathy, and many dozens of homeopathic hospitals

- The prefix, "homeo" means similar or the same. The suffix, "pathy" refers to feeling, symptoms, suffering, disease, or illness.

- Today, homeopathy is used by millions of people in more than 65 countries, and over 400,000 health care professionals. It is an internationally-accepted natural therapeutic approach.

- England's royal family has used and advocated homeopathy non-stop since it was first established. Her Majesty, Queen Elizabeth II and Prince Charles are avid supporters of homeopathy, as was Princess Diana. The Queen has benefited from the services of the *Royal London Homeopathic Hospital*. The Queen Mother, who lived to age 101, was the principal patron of the *British Homeopathic Association*.

- Several U.S. presidents used homeopathy, as do many prominent wealthy celebrities and elite athletes. This is important because these people can afford *any* medical care, and by choice they include homeopathy.

- The *National Center for Complementary and Alternative Medicine* (NCCAM)—a U.S. government agency, classifies homeopathy as a whole medical system.

- Homeopathy has been approved and strictly regulated by the FDA since 1938.

- The "father" of modern homeopathy, Dr. Samuel Hahnemann has been immortalized in statue at Scott Circle in Washington D.C. He was the respected German physician, whose awareness of the dangers of pharmaceutical medicine prompted him to find a safer approach.

- Positive research studies have been published in medical journals—including one from through *M.D. Anderson Cancer Research Center*, published in the *International Journal of Oncology*.

- The roots of homeopathy date back to Hippocrates— the "father of modern medicine" (460 BC – 370 BC) in Greece. They were furthered by Renaissance physician, Paracelsus (1493-1541) in Switzerland.

- Homeopathic remedies are NOT herbal medicines. Homeopathic remedies are derived from some plant sources, but also from animal, and mineral sources.

- Homeopathy is a form of energy medicine. Remedies do not contain any pharmacologically active substances, nor do they produce any chemical action or reaction.

- Homeopathic remedies are safe and fully-compatible with any other medical treatment, including prescription drugs. They have no known side effects or drug interactions.

- Pharmaceutical medicine involves highly concentrated forms of various substances. In essence, homeopathic medicine is the exact *opposite* approach. Doctors throughout the world were attracted to homeopathy during the early 1800s.

- Homeopathy is not addictive, and it works in harmony with your immune system, rather than suppressing symptoms.

- Homeopathic medicine focuses on the symptoms of the *individual*, rather than those of a specific medical condition. It is intended to treat the person with the illness, rather than the illness as the entity.

- Homeopathy is intended to support the body's inborn healing capacity by introducing to the body bio-energetic (rather than bio-chemical) stimuli that are similar to the symptoms of the illness itself. This appears to trigger the body to take more aggressive action towards healing itself from within.

- The homeopathic approach takes into account the whole person, including the patient's entire emotional, general, and physical condition, as well as minute details not typically considered by most doctors.

- Since homeopathy is a whole person approach, the treatments selected are often completely different for each person—even if they have the same symptoms or medically diagnosed condition as another.

More accurately, homeopathy is solely a *treatment* system because it does not involve medical diagnosis. If this seems peculiar, consider that pharmaceutical medications are rampantly prescribed to treat symptoms—even when no formal diagnosis has been made. There is however, a huge difference. With homeopathy, we are not treating the symptoms, but rather the PERSON who suffers the symptoms.

What Hippocrates Knew
That Most Doctors Have Forgotten

With Western pharmaceutical medicine, chemical drugs are administered to create an opposite effect of the patient's symptoms. For example, antacids are given for digestive problems, antidepressants for depression, antihistamines for allergies, etc. With homeopathy, it is quite the contrary. The main principle of homeopathy is known as the *Law of Similars*.

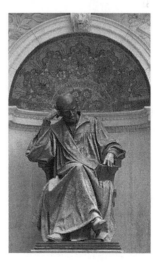

Here's what it's all about:

Imagine a substance, such as a plant root. A healthy person eats some of it, and develops symptoms similar to a particular known medical ailment. This same substance could also be

185

utilized to help a person suffering the actual ailment! How? If a small sample of our hypothetical root were meticulously diluted over and over (and violently shaken in between each dilution) such that no molecules of the original physical substance existed anymore in the solution, a homeopathic remedy would be the result. This remedy would no longer possess chemical attributes, nor would any pharmaceutically active substance exist in the solution. However, what *would* be left in the solution is the electromagnetic frequency or energetic "footprint" of the original substance. It appears that exposure to the energetic frequencies or imprint of the original substance can result in an ailing body receiving an "extra push," to recover from the disease itself from within, by means of the person's immune system.

This is precisely how German physician, **Dr. Samuel Hahnemann** "re-discovered" and refined the medical principles laid down by Hippocrates (Greece, 470-400 B.C.), the "Father of Medicine." Dr. Hahnemann felt that the medicines of his time did as much harm as good. Medical use of mercury and arsenic were commonplace, prompting his desire for safer treatments. Hahnemann was an advocate of patients getting plenty of fresh air and sunshine, rest, proper diet, good hygiene and various other natural health measures. This was during a time in history when other physicians considered these practices to be *ridiculous!* Physicians such as Hippocrates, Paracelsus, Hahnemann, Nogier, and Soliman laid the foundation for those willing to be unconventional—to really make a difference for sick and suffering people.

Barking up the <u>Right</u> Tree

Hahnemann's famous experiment involved Peruvian Cinchona bark from which quinine, the treatment for malaria was derived. He found that small doses of whole Cinchona given to a *healthy* person would cause symptoms similar to malaria. He later

186

discovered that much smaller and diluted doses (violently shaken between dilutions) would produce an effective remedy. It provided a safe and gentle stimulus to help a malaria victim naturally get better. Such effect was not rendered by chemical medicinal action, but rather the patient's own inborn healing capacity! He used a substance that caused a similar feeling or symptoms of an illness (in its whole form) to treat a person with the actual illness (in its highly-diluted form). Dr. Hahneman reintroduced this as the working principle of homeopathy, originally championed by Hippocrates and Paracelsus.

Conventional Western medicine is based on a bio-*chemical* health care philosophy, where *concentrated* substances are administered in *large* doses. By contrast homeopathic remedies have no chemical action whatsoever. They are NOT prescription drugs. Homeopathy is a bio-*energetic* approach, where highly *diluted* substances are administered in infinitesimally *small* doses. For example a remedy may by one part of the substance in 1,000,000,000,000 parts water. This is indeed a principle not fully understood or agreed upon scientifically, however the clinical results support the hypothesis.

Here are some simple examples:

- Epsom salts (Magnesium Sulphate) may be given to a person to help constipation. But a homeopathic remedy derived from Magnesium Sulphate can help relieve *diarrhea!*

- Drinking coffee can stimulate your nervous system and keep you awake, causing insomnia. But a homeopathic remedy derived from coffee can help calm the nervous system and promote natural sleep.

- Did you ever get watery, burning, or itchy eyes when peeling onions? Maybe you'll also get a runny, drippy nose—like when you have a cold too. A homeopathically diluted preparation of red onion (*Allium cepa*) can be taken to help your body heal itself from a cold (or just chronically drippy eyes). The homeopathic dilution formula created originally from an onion has the *reverse* effect on the body: it helps with the very symptoms a whole onion would *cause*.

A homeopathy-based evaluation tends to take much longer than most conventional medical exams. Much more detail is sought. For example, one would not simply tell the doctor "I have headaches" and be prescribed a remedy in the manner that one would be prescribed the latest prescription headache medicine. It is not "one size fits all" treatment. With dozens of potential causes of chronic headaches, the homeopathic support will differ from person to person.

FACT: Homeopathy is NOT Herbal Medicine!

Homeopathy is frequently confused with herbal medicine. Perhaps this stems from the fact that many homeopathic remedies have their origins with herbs and other plants. However, homeopathic remedies are also derived from nearly any substance found in nature, including animal and mineral sources. Homeopathic remedies and herbal medicines are created, and act by completely different mechanisms. Herbal medicines operate in basically the same manner as pharmaceutical medicines—through bio-**chemical** action. Chemical reactions from herbal substances, like laboratory-synthesized drugs, suppress symptoms by speeding up or slowing down chemical processes in the body.

By contrast, homeopathy is bio-**energetic** medicine. There is no chemical effect whatsoever—a concept new to most people, although nothing *new* at all. Homeopathy works by means of resonant frequencies of substances that support body function. A homeopathic remedy "nags" the body to have a stronger response and become more efficient. Homeopathy naturally supports the defensive mechanisms of the human body to take a more aggressive action *itself* against the various causes of the illness and pain. Unlike both the drugs of conventional Western medicine and herbal medications, homeopathy lacks any side effects and complications.

Herbal medicine certainly has its place in the health care. It is not however, part of the *Bio-energetic Individualized Therapy Equation*. Although I have professional access to herbs for my patients, I choose not to use them for various reasons. In my experience, the homeopathic approach works better, and blows herbal medicine away in terms of safety. The quality of homeopathic remedies is FDA regulated. The homeopathic pharmacopoeia of the United States was written into federal law in 1938 under the *Federal Food, Drug, and Cosmetic Act*. Herbal products, which can cause side effects and drug interactions, are *not* regulated. Herbal medications come from nature rather than a laboratory, but that does not make them automatically safe.

"If Homeopathy is So Wonderful, Why is it NOT Part of American Mainstream Medicine?"

Homeopathy was once an integral part of America medical care, and was taught in many prestigious medical schools. It has been continuously maintained as an accepted component of many effective health care systems throughout the world for over 200 years. Homeopathy was introduced to America in 1824, and the *American Institute of Homeopathy* was founded in 1844. Unfortunately, this came at a time when the burgeoning pharmaceutical-based medicine establishment was showing unyielding intolerance and animosity towards *any* competition. The *American Medical Association* (AMA) was founded in 1847, largely to annihilate homeopathy! Sadly, by 1925, homeopathy was driven to extinction in America. When Rockefeller and Carnegie donated huge amounts of money to develop AMA medicine, homeopathy was destroyed to pave the way for the highly-lucrative drug-based medicine.

In the chapter on bio-electric fields, you learned that the commissioning of the *Flexner Report* resulted in medical schools becoming drug-based institutions. There had been many schools teaching a great diversity of health care methods. The horrifying but successful business strategy of the "founding fathers" of "Big Pharma" was to blatantly eliminate *anything* outside the realm of drug-based medicine. The AMA prohibited membership from their professional organization, and ostracized any doctors who practiced homeopathy. The subtle, gradual, and natural approach of homeopathy was eclipsed by the "magic bullet" concept developing in the pharmaceutical field. Drugs could be patented and become investment commodities, which added to their corporate business pedigree. Homeopathic remedies and other supplements are not patentable.

The criticism that the mechanism of homeopathy is unknown, or that it "couldn't work" is laughable at best. We can add it to the many mysteries of nature not yet understood. It wasn't until 1995 that science provided a more detailed explanation of how aspirin works. Good thing we didn't wait for this explanation!

Clearly the mechanisms of homeopathy are not simple, nor are they easy and quick to understand. Bear in mind that this is equally or further the case with regards to comprehension of the biochemistry and physiological actions of conventional prescription medicine. It is unknown to scientists how *many* FDA-approved drugs work.

"The health problems I was having when I first came in were: spacey/dizziness, left upper quadrant and rib pain, headaches, hot flashes and night sweats, liver dysfunction, gastrointestinal dysfunction, body or bony pain, irritability and sensitivity to light and noise, memory problems like dyslexia, forgetfulness, and word recall, and shakiness. I had "chronic fatigue" and in the beginning had mono for nine months after diagnosis. I was too tired to get out of bed any earlier that 10 or 11 am. I was sleeping away most of my day. The noise of my job would make me angry. The quick action type work that I have was affected by my memory problems... My personal life was also affected. I was too tired to do anything. I felt like there was no hope for getting rid of this disease. I was going to specialist and they told me they could not help me or that because I took antibiotics I was cured. I was getting very depressed and hopeless. Angry that no one could help and very angry at the cost of the people who thought said they could.

I could not do my job the right way. I missed many days from work for the simple fact I could not get out of bed. I am a runner and hiker and I could not do the activities I enjoyed so much. Taking my beautiful dog on a walk around the neighborhood was taxing. I had to watch everything I ate because I never knew what was going to make me sick. I didn't eat at my own wedding because I was afraid I would get sick because of the gastro problems I was having. We didn't' go out as much because I would feel so run down. I tried antibiotics from my GP on multiple occasions, I went to three infectious disease doctors who all told me the same thing "no such thing as chronic Lyme, you are cured—you took antibiotics, don't know what is wrong with you". I was checked for MS from a neurologist, I was checked for Chron's and Celiac from a gastroenterologist, I went out to a treatment center in Arizona who took a more natural supplement approach to Lyme and had great success, but it was short lived and very expensive.

I really don't have any symptoms, and have had no problem or side effects from the [BITE] treatment. My quality of life has improved 100%... I feel human again. I can do my job, go out with my husband, and the best thing is being pregnant with my first child and not worry about harming them or lying in bed all day. I can go out on walks and get up before 10 am in the

191

morning which is a big deal. When you sleep all day you feel like there is nothing to live for but sleep. When you can get up a decent time and do something with your day, it feels wonderful.

Dr. Liebell and his staff are down to earth people who are happy to see you when you come in. Listen to what you have to say without making judgment and with an open mind. They have been through the same agony and understand what and how you feel. They understand the frustrations of not being able to fix a problem. They are not out to make money but to help you feel good again. Testing is painless and quick. You don't feel anything at all. What can I say, what do you have to lose? I have taken many rounds of antibiotics and tried other extremely expensive treatments. This is the most effective thing I have done for this disease. With the results that you get, you can't go wrong. I went almost three years without knowing if I would ever beat this. I had one doctor tell me I would have Lyme for the rest of my life and all I could do was manage my symptoms. With this treatment there was hope of beating it and living a normal healthy, pain free life. I only wish I would have found Dr. Liebell earlier in my struggle with Lyme."

- Amanda M., Williamsburg, VA

An American Homeopathic Renaissance

Fortunately, by the 1970s, homeopathy began its American comeback as people started to become aware of natural foods, exercise and the effects of pollution and environmental toxins. Today, homeopathy is used worldwide with expanding popularity. Over the past 15 years or so, advancements have been made in Europe, gradually filtering into the United States. Americans want safe, effective, and affordable health care. It certainly appears that we are literally sick and tired of a system that pushes drugs and surgery first, with an insurance system that denies many cost-effective, natural and preventative methods. Thus, homeopathy has become "re-discovered" in recent years. Further upgrades in technology have advanced it as

192

well. These advancements were responsible for my wife, Sheila to overcome chronic tick-triggered illness, thus propelling me to re-invent my practice to help others likewise.

If you are interested in looking up and learning about homeopathic remedies listed in the Homeopathic Pharmacopeia of the United States (HPUS), you have access to various online resources:

- http://www.hpus.com/
- http://hpathy.com/materia-medica/
- http://www.vithoulkas.com/en/books-study/online-materia-medica.html
- http://hpathy.com/scientific-research/

'I'm looking for a lot of men who have an infinite capacity to not know what can't be done.' — Henry Ford

Chapter 25:

Bio-energetic Wellness Supplementation

Authentic natural healthcare is not merely using products from nature, nor does it simply mean drug-free treatment. Lots of substances are technically natural; it does not mean they have medicinal value, nor can we assume their safety. By its strictest definition, natural healthcare includes methods which support the body to regulate and repair itself, through its own inborn (natural) mechanisms. BITE methods fit this description precisely. Bio-energetic supplementation is one such approach, which has supported patients to naturally overcome a wide variety of health problems. They work based upon time-tested holistic wellness principles (inspired by homeopathy), combined with modern technology. However, they are not multi-vitamin supplements, nor are they herbal medicines or oils. They are formulated based upon bio-energetic, rather than bio-chemical principles. We have all been raised with the bio-chemical model of medicine—so it can take some effort, time, and repetitive explanation to grasp bio-energetics.

Clinically, Lyme disease is a classic example of the individual nature of human response to one particular agent of disease. The *Borrelia burgdorferi* bacterium is the same, but the variation in symptoms for each person infected by it is astonishing. One person may become afflicted with migraines, yet others might develop Bell's palsy, multiple sclerosis, POTS disease, or peripheral neuropathy. Some victims suffer heart problems, while others infected by the same microbe only experience chronic joint pain. Still others develop symptoms diagnosed as fibromyalgia. This is why the bio-energetic holistic wellness approach revolves around the *person* rather than the disease!

Mainstream medicine tends to view patients as medical *conditions* rather than unique people. One of the key factors for helping people recover from tick-triggered illness is treating each person individually. There is no set "Lyme protocol." I have reinforced throughout this book that the BITE is not a treatment for Lyme disease. It is administered and intended solely as wellness support. Each patient's individualized treatment is determined beginning with data collected from filling out medical health history forms. This is followed by a comprehensive and lengthy consultation—to get all the details about the person. This goes far and beyond merely learning about current symptoms or any previous medical diagnosis. The most obscure little details about a person can be extremely helpful for the doctor to determine effective supportive holistic treatment. One's medical history *prior* to apparent tick-borne infection is often just as important—if not more so than current and recent symptoms. For example, many patients report having suffered mononucleosis ("mono") years or decades prior to Lyme infection. The Epstein-Barr virus associated with the condition can lurk silently in one's body awaiting the opportunity to thrive due to a malfunctioning immune system. "Chronic fatigue syndrome" may be the result (recently renamed myalgic encephalomyelitis, and then changed to systemic exertion intolerance disease)!). This is of course, another reminder of why it is illogical to expect to overcome chronic illness through long-term antibiotic usage. Thorough case history often points to numerous non-bacterial causes of chronic pain and illness.

It takes considerable time, patience, thoughtfulness, and skill to provide effective bio-energetic supplementation treatment. The process is quite different from merely prescribing drugs or other

195

treatments that match up with a "one-size-fits-all" medical diagnosis. There is no standard bio-energetic supplement protocol for any one condition. Ten people could have the same symptoms—each requiring a completely *different* support regimen. Once a thorough health history and consultation is complete, bio-energetic testing is performed. The combination of these approaches leads the doctor to perform any appropriate auricular therapy, and to generate the patient's individualized bio-energetic supplement protocol.

Life is Energy in Motion

The term "bio-energetic" means *living energy*. The proprietary bio-energetic supplements we utilize are the ultimate part of the *Bio-energetic Individual Treatment Equation*©. Each patient's customized regimen includes between five and fifteen different bio-energetic support "formulas" that work together as a whole. How these supplements are created, and how they work are both extremely complex matters, which admittedly are not yet fully understood scientifically. Nevertheless, the results my family and my patients have achieved through their usage has been phenomenal, to say the least. I am not a physicist, nor do I require or expect my patients to understand the mechanisms of product creation. What I am providing for you here is some fundamental background.

Bio-energetic Supplementation

The proprietary bio-energetic supplements used by BITE practitioners are encoded liquids. They are custom created for us by a sophisticated process of embedding virtual blueprints of substances. These are called **informational imprints**. The process of creating an informational imprint was introduced around 2007. Precise multi-layered images of the desired substance (for energetic simulation) are created from symbols, shapes and colors. They are interwoven with alpha-numeric characters, which may be up to 300,000 pages long. These signatures are then converted to a digitally-formatted card. This process is called *Coherent Energy Transduction*. To create the liquid sublingual spray supplements, the card is placed in an instrument called an *Alpha-numeric Transducer* (ANT). The ANT imprints the energetic signatures into a liquid solution of water, a miniscule amount of pure organic alcohol (less than 0.0017 ounce per spray), and a few trace minerals.

Different products are created by embedding specific encoded data into a blank solution. Each one is composed of many dozens of different encoded informational imprints, crafted from a constantly expanding database. **The informational imprints are** <u>replicas</u> **of a wide variety of substances from plants, animals, minerals, vitamins, amino acids, and other natural sources.** This includes informational imprints replicating the signals of several thousand long-established natural remedies. **However, no actual physical substances are ever used**.

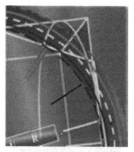

*Dynamic Encoding
Image of Sulphur*

Does the concept of encoding water with informational imprints sound far-fetched or outrageous?

Encoded water is as comprehensible as many long-established technologies. Consider how music records have been made,

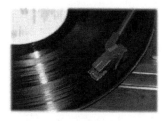

dating back to Thomas Edison's first phonograph. Vibration patterns are etched by a stylus into the blank record during live sound recording. The master imprint gets processed, and duplicates can be made. The sound can be played back by the

197

phonograph's player's needle sitting in the record's groove, which contains the preserved energy pattern of the original sound. Amazing!

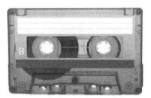

With audio or videotape, complex data is stored *magnetically* on iron coated plastic tape (can you believe that this is *old* technology?). **Modern CDs and DVDs store information optically, embedded into a piece of polycarbonate plastic.** With usage, laser beams detect embedded coding of numbers, spaces and microscopic bumps. Quite frankly, vinyl records and magnetic tape seem easier to understand!

DVDs bring us the complexities of motion, color, and sound to our televisions and computers. A blank disc can have infinite combinations of digital data encoded into it. This determines what movie, music, or other computer data can be accessed and utilized.

Scientists have developed many astonishing ways to capture and utilize energy patterns. Much of what was once considered science fiction has been surpassed by scientific reality. We open car doors with keypads projecting frequencies specific to our own vehicle. A radio can be tuned to a specific frequency. We transmit messages, data, video, photos, and voice around the world, instantly via smart phones. We can use Skype or Facetime, and stream Netflix to our televisions and phones. There are so many astonishing ways that scientists have enabled us to transmit and store signals, instantly. Quite frankly, the idea of informational imprints embedded in water supporting our health seems comparatively simple in comparison! Bio-energetic supplements are created by embedding signals into water.

Water Memory

The term used by Nobel Prize-winning scientist Dr. Luc Montagnier is <u>water memory</u>. Montagnier has declared that DNA emits electromagnetic waves that can be retained in water. He confirmed the hypothesis that water can retain the frequencies, imprints, or energetic signatures of substances. Dr. Montagnier won the 2008 Nobel Prize for discovery of the AIDS virus (HIV).

Dr. Montagnier also verified that the electromagnetic signals retained in water can have dramatic *biological* effects! Unfortunately some of Dr. Montagnier's peers do not get it. Oddly, many have criticized his water research because its mechanisms are not yet fully understood. Isn't investigation and discovery the purpose of scientific research? It is peculiar how much energy and time has been spent throughout history criticizing anything different from established and old ways.

> *"Discovery consists of looking at the same thing as everyone else and thinking something different"*
>
> -Albert Szent-Gyorgi (Nobel Prize winning biochemist)

My patients, family, friends, and I are quite certain that water memory and the beneficial physiological effects of informational imprints have propelled them towards better health. So, if your local MD doesn't believe it, perhaps you might put more trust in the opinion of a world-renowned scientist. In his 2010 interview with *Science Magazine*, Dr. Montagnier reminded readers of the impressive results of similar remedies (homeopathic) during the nineteenth century with epidemics of cholera, typhoid, yellow fever, scarlet fever, and influenza. The professor has declared that water structures can mimic molecules of substances—without any physical substance present. Montagnier plans on continuing research on the phenomenon of electromagnetic waves produced by DNA in water—in particular the DNA of bacteria and viruses, and its impact on treatment of chronic disease. Dr. Montagnier has pointed out however, that funding for research will be scarce since the conventional pharmaceutical companies cannot benefit from furthering drug-free treatments. Luc Montagnier is a medical doctor. He is certain that the principle of water memory brings tremendous research opportunity for modern medicine. Dr. Montagnier has moved to China to continue his research.

Here's a link to an interesting documentary film about Dr. Luc Montagnier's water memory research. He shows how virus DNA signal can be captured in water, recorded, and transmitted as a computer file:
https://www.youtube.com/watch?v=R8VyUsVOic0

Dr. James Oschman, another world-renowned scientist holds the same view about water. He is a physiologist, cellular biologist, and biophysicist. Dr. Oschman is the most prominent academic scientist to explore the basis for natural and holistic therapies. He has published dozens of articles in academic scientific journals. Dr. Oschman references that the same scientific methods that have been utilized to provide the basis for *conventional* chemical medical practice have been used equally to evaluate energy medicine.

According to Oschman, in his book *"Energy Medicine—the Scientific Basis"* the principle of water memory does *not* violate any known laws of physics or nature (as some naysayers insist). He indicates that this is the thinking of scientists from ten different nations. Oschman acknowledges that our scientific understanding of the physics of water is incomplete. He has described the human body as a living crystal with electricity, magnetism, and light flowing through it, often at higher speeds than the standard neurology model. Dr. Oschman's book is a fantastic resource. It shows how bio-energetic science can be used to help people overcome illnesses, which have responded poorly to pharmaceutical medicine. It provides a deep understanding about energy and energy flow in the human body, with well-established and documented scientific research. He describes how various methods can restore natural energy flow within the body, which supports recovery from many problems.

Another Nobel Prize-winning scientist, Brian Josephson, Ph.D. is a supporter of homeopathic medicine. In an article in *New Scientist*, Dr. Josephson defended the common criticism that homeopathy "couldn't work" since there are no molecules of other substances present in the water. This Cambridge University physics professor reminded naysayers that the beneficial effects of homeopathy have *never* been claimed to be due to the presence of molecules of medicinal substances, but rather the water's structure, which contains embedded energy imprints. Like many things used in *conventional* medicine, it is not yet fully understood to science how encoding water with informational imprints facilitates the clinically-observed health improvements. What my family, my patients, and I know for sure is that bio-energetic supplementation absolutely does work! The principle of embedding energy signals into water described by these Nobel Laureates is the mechanism behind the bio-energetic supplement products I recommend and personally use.

The water and its embedded informational imprints do not treat any symptom or medical condition. However, the clinical results suggest that their usage clearly encourages people's bodies to do what they're naturally supposed to do, when for whatever reasons, function has been suppressed. Clinical results suggest consistent daily exposure to their beneficial frequencies results in the ailing and struggling body developing a heightened sense of its existing problems. It seems clear that this serves as a safe and gentle "push" for the body to work harder itself to get better through its own inborn physiological mechanisms.

It is a scientific fact that people can naturally acquire better functional immunity, and improve their health by their bodies own internal inborn mechanisms. Some people never catch colds, regardless of their exposure to sick people. Others never succumb to the flu or other viruses and other germs spreading around a community. They are fortunate to have strong immunity towards *those* particular germs. For example, some people are immune to the infectious microbes transmitted by tick bites; they do not develop Lyme disease. Others are not so fortunate, and need help.

A Symphony of Support

It is well-known that music can have beneficial physiological effects. Imagine a symphony orchestra playing a specific musical chord. Imagine a violinist plays a certain note. The harpist plans another. The pianist strikes a complex chord with all ten fingers. The percussionist crashes the cymbals, while the clarinet, oboe, and trombonist all play different notes too. Each musician contributes a vibrational frequency to create the synchronized whole musical unit.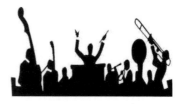

Each bio-energetic supplement is embedded with informational imprints each of which have a distinct role or function—like different notes being played by a variety of different musical instruments in a symphony orchestra. This is what each bio-energetic supplement is meant to do: create a symphony of signals. When you take a spray, think of it like a symphony orchestra striking a specific chord, with each musician producing musical tones of a distinct vibrational frequency. Each time a bio-energetic product is sprayed under the tongue, you receive a burst of the beneficial "harmonies" of its specific combination of informational imprints. Each individual product is like a music CD; the plastic disc is identical for every music recording, but the embedded digital coding of the music recording is different. Each distinct bio-energetic supplement "plays a different chord." The cumulative effect of the different chords from each supplement taking in succession produces the "song."

Daily regular usage provides the whole-body, holistic wellness support. The doctor's job is to figure out what "chords" each person needs to produce the right "song" for each patient. This is obviously not a rigid protocol for any particular medical condition, nor is it the same for every patient. Although they do not treat any medical condition directly; every bio-energetic supplement has a unique combination of informational imprints for specific purposes. There are supports for specific organs and tissues such as the liver, kidneys, adrenal glands, brain, muscles, tendons, nerves, etc. Others serve to aid cellular detoxification or natural support for one's natural physiology to deal with pathogens and parasites, solar and geomagnetic activity, and metal toxicity. What products are chosen depends upon the needs of the individual.

<u>**The bottles do not list the informational imprints.**</u> There are several reasons for this. For starters, there are too many to fit on the labels; some products have hundreds of them. Facsimiles or energetic representations of signals of thousands of natural substances can be used. Each product is like a music CD; the blank plastic disc is identical for every music recording, but the embedded digital coding of the music recording is different and unique for each. Having a list of the informational imprints would be sort of like printing the written musical score of a music CD on the disc label.

Bio-energetic supplements are classified and regulated as dietary supplements. It is required by law that only the water, mineral, and alcohol—the *physical* ingredients must be listed on product labels. The various products have different names (and purposes), but the liquid solution's ingredients are always the same. Each product has a unique combination of embedded informational imprints. Listing all of each product's specific informational imprints is neither required, nor feasible. This is like "natural flavors" listed as an ingredient on food product labels. Thousands of possible chemical substances extracted from plant or animal sources are used. A food product may contain natural flavoring composed of as many as 100 different substances. They are not listed, nor does the U.S. Code of Federal Regulations require it. Natural flavoring is not considered nutritional. It would not be feasible to list such components on labels. The same is the case for bio-energetic supplements.

These are proprietary formulas that have taken years of study, effort, and tens of thousands of dollars to research and develop. Unlike pharmaceutical drugs, bio-energetic supplement formulas cannot be patented or publicly traded on the stock exchange. The informational imprint component formulas are however, intellectual property, like a book's copyright or a secret formula. They are not for public distribution. If they were made public; they could be easily copied, stolen, and illegally used. Upon request, I can show you, or verbally describe some of them. They are mostly in Latin scientific terminology. All patients use bio-energetic supplements must do so with the understanding, acceptance, and trust that they are embedded with different combinations of informational imprints. Bio-energetic supplements are never represented as having any pharmaceutical action, nor are they suggested as treatment of any medical condition, in the conventional sense.

Key Points Regarding
Bio-energetic Supplements:

It appears that with bio-energetic support, patients are developing their own natural immunity, which enables their bodies to better deal with stressors that result in pain and illness. Let me be crystal clear that this is not a medical claim; we currently have no academic scientific proof. However, the response patients demonstrate and report suggests this is the case.

The dynamic effects of bio-energetic supplements are solely the result of your body's natural and normal physiological mechanisms. The intention of bio-energetic support is to fortify your body's awareness of its existing problems, so it acts more aggressively to improve itself, naturally.

Unlike chemical pharmaceutical drugs (and some herbal products), our bio-energetic supplements <u>cannot</u> and do not make your body do *anything* that it is not physiologically supposed to do.

Each spray of a bio-energetic supplement delivers a burst of complex informational imprints, which simulate various supportive substances. This is intended to serve as a stimulus to the body to "remind" it to carry out its own natural self-regulating processes, which are stagnated or "stuck."

These products deliver NO chemical pharmaceutical effects, nor are they addictive. They are safe and compatible for use with <u>any</u> other treatments, supplements, foods, as well as pharmaceutical medications provided by other physicians.

Our bio-energetic supplements are NOT drugs, nor are they controlled substances. They cannot and do not cause chemical side effects, nor is there any concern for drug interactions with pharmaceutical medication (or <u>anything</u> else you may be taking, eating, or doing).

Bio-energetic supplements are NOT herbs, nor do the bear any resemblance to them in form or function. Herbal medicines work by means of <u>chemical</u> action, and are very similar to pharmaceutical medications. Herbs are the raw materials for many drugs.

There is NO measurable chemically medicinal substance in our bio-energetic products. The physical ingredients are the <u>same</u> liquid solution for each product. However, the complex <u>bio-energetic encoding</u> is completely different for each. The nutrient ingredient is malic acid, in a tiny amount. Malic acid is a beneficial component of various fruits.

The working principle of the bio-energetic supplements is _water memory_. This is the terminology of Nobel Prize-winning scientist Dr. Luc Montagnier. Montagnier determined that DNA emits electromagnetic waves that can be retained in water. He confirmed that water can retain the frequencies, imprints, or energetic signatures of substances. Such signals can have dramatic _biological_ effects!

Our bio-energetic supplements are liquid solutions that have been embedded with formulated code. A CD or DVD is a piece of plastic with digital code embedded within it. Similarly, each bio-energetic supplement product is a precisely encoded liquid with different specific components.

These products do not contain any substance that could or would provoke a toxic response. This includes a very insignificant amount of pure organic alcohol (0.0017 ounce per spray). An average protocol composed of 12 sprays delivers a miniscule total of 0.02 ounces of alcohol (that's two one hundreds of one ounce, one tenth of a teaspoon). The aerosol effect of the pump sprayer does tend to magnify the alcohol smell and taste; however, it is an extremely small amount of alcohol. The only consideration is if a person is known to be *allergic* to alcohol. Many prescription and over-the-counter medicines contain significant amounts of alcohol, as well as some foods.

None of these bio-energetic supplements are represented, suggested, claimed, or intended to prevent or treat any specific medical condition, nor are they intended to replace or delay any necessary conventional medical care. They are intended solely to support one's natural inborn physiological regulation.

I claim no proof of any specific physiological mechanism beyond the fact of clinical improvements reported by patients and where physically possible, observed.

These products are not commercial stock items; they cannot be purchased at a health food store or online. They are manufactured for us upon demand, and are constantly updated and improved as well.

Here's how an initial daily bio-energetic wellness regimen is done:

Each patient's customized daily protocol includes as many as fifteen different support products that <u>work together as a whole</u>. Each product is sprayed just once under the tongue, one after another. The order in which they are taken does not matter, nor must a strict timetable be followed. The entire process takes a minute or less, initially done three times daily, for the first two months. Whatever times of day that are convenient for you are fine. Leave at least one hour in between.

There's nothing to think about, otherwise. There's no swishing it around in your mouth or counting how many seconds to hold the liquid before swallowing. No contemplating or questioning. Just spray, and go about your day! This is not the same as taking a pill, and waiting for its effects to kick in. This is supplying your body with a bio-energetic "reminder" of the critically important and complex job it must do to get healthier. The trace amount of malic acid is the beneficial supplemental nutrient in each spray.

I cannot stress it enough that bio-energetic supplementation does not, and cannot make your body do anything it should not (or could not) do naturally. The translation of that: NO side effects.

The specific individual bio-energetic products in each patient's customized wellness protocol combine to function as ONE synchronized cohesive functioning unit—a whole-body support. They should not be viewed as individual *medicines* (they are not drugs).

All protocol component products are included specifically because the doctor determines through bio-energetic testing that you will likely benefit from them. A baker would never bake a cake, intentionally leave out one or more key ingredients… and expect the cake to come out right. An orchestra would not play Beethoven's fifth symphony without the violin section and the horns. Similarly, with a bio-energetic supplement protocols, patients should resist any temptation to use only *some* of your recommended products thinking that (for some reason), all are not needed. The same is the case for using all of the recommended products, at the frequency listed for each (3x/day, 2x/day, 1x/day, or 1x/week).

It's quite simple: patients who follow their individualized protocol correctly get the best results.

208

The *Bio-energetic Individual Treatment Equation©* (BITE) is not a replacement for conventional medical care. It is a holistic wellness support program. In no manner whatsoever is it a treatment for any disease by strict medical definition. Have I mentioned this a few times before? Repetition is well-needed!

"I was nervous about the Auricular therapy... however I immediately felt a "whoosh" and temporary dizziness. I felt immediately better; my sinuses opened and I felt energized. The following week my energy level went thru the roof. I am strong and do not need pain medication anymore. The [bio-energetic] formulations were easy to use... Within a few weeks I began to feel my legs and could walk and stand longer and my digestive tract became normal. I have become more mobile and have dropped 70 pounds. I am a year out and last Sunday I walked, yes walked at Busch Gardens from noon until 10pm without difficulty. My friends wore out faster than me. Woo-Hoo! I feel I am living life again! Praise God for Dr. Liebell.
–Regina C., PhD., Virginia Beach

"I had no quality of life...at times I would consider suicide. My life was spent in the bed almost 24/7. I was given all types of antibiotics. I was diagnosed with MS and given medication. Later they decided I had Fibromyalgia—now different medication... and nothing worked. I also had countless blood tests, MRIs, and Cat Scans which showed nothing abnormal. I had one doctor even send me to a shrink, that didn't work either. When I was at my worst I was terminated from my employer...for being sick.

I had the [bio-energetic] testing and the treatments.... You don't feel a thing ...the easiest testing I have ever had. The homeopathic supplements are easy to take and affordable too—a lot cheaper than medication and without the side effects! The ear acupuncture treatment is simple... just a little pressure and it works. I had things that other doctors did that hurt me and didn't work either. The improvements I have received from Dr. Liebell are FABULOUS. I have my life back... Who knew it could be so simple and to think how much I suffered needlessly. MY LIFE IS WONDERFUL!!!! I can do anything and everything I want. Life is good!!! Dr. Liebell and his staff are incredible...they listen and, they are always there to help. He is one in a million. People who think antibiotics are their only hope need to give this a try... they don't have anything to lose. Not only did I have Lyme disease, but I had a few other issues also that needed to be treated. I personally guarantee they will feel better than they ever did, and they have a doctor that actually gives a damn!"

- Karen S., Windsor, VA

"I had been diagnosed with late stage Lyme - at least two years of infection. The bulk of my escalating issues were digestive, joint and cognitive. I truly thought I would no longer be able to function professionally. Unable to move, unable to think, had a negative spiral effect on me...lowered self-esteem, depression, sadness, and isolation. I was unable to engage in simple daily activities like climbing stairs. Getting up from a chair was often a struggle. Getting on the treadmill was out of the question. My knuckles hurt so bad that sometimes I couldn't sleep at night. And my memory felt like it was melting away. My medical path took me initially to my physician's assistant, who referred me to several specialists, e.g., osteoarthritis doctors, psychiatrist, orthopedics, gastrointestinal, and lots of lab and x-ray visits. I no longer was surprised with having 12 vials of blood drawn.

There is no way for me to quantify my peace of mind. I'm returning to my former self (ok, I'm a little older now). But the ability to move, think, and ingest has returned, not to mention the ENERGY! Wahoo! I am now able to re-focus on personal, professional, and academic goals that I thought I was going to have to abandon. It's like getting a new lease on life - that probably sounds hokey, but it's true! I want you to picture a middle-aged woman doing cartwheels down the aisle...that's me! For chronic Lyme sufferers, who don't believe that any treatment other than antibiotics could be a solution: How badly do you want your life back???"

- Donna Z., PhD, Glen Allen, VA

People are Absolutely Capable of Getting Well

Some people never catch colds, regardless of their exposure to sick people. Others never succumb to the flu or other "bugs" going around in the community. They are fortunate to have strong immunity towards those particular germs. The fact is some people are *immune* to the *Borrelia* bacteria of Lyme disease too. They can be bitten by infectious ticks, but <u>not</u> develop Lyme disease. It stands to reason that one can *develop* immunity to it as well. It appears that with the *Bio-energetic Individual Treatment Equation*©, patients are developing natural immunity. Let me be clear that this is not a medical claim; we have no academic scientific proof of this at this point in time. However, the response patients demonstrate and report suggests this is the case.

It is necessary for me to clarify that this book has primarily been written as a resource for people who are certain their health has been deteriorated by tick-borne infection. This does not mean that a doctor has diagnosed Lyme disease, nor does it matter whether or not it is the case. When people suffer symptoms for which no cause-related diagnosis is ever provided, they will mostly receive treatment that in no way addresses or affects the causes of the problems. I humbly state that people seek my care because they have failed to improve despite multiple efforts from multiple doctors and other health practitioners. Our holistic bio-energetic wellness approach is for those who have failed to get well despite being assured no active infection exists in their bodies. It is for those who have been told they have been "cured" of Lyme disease and any well-known tick-borne co-infections because they have taken antibiotics, and blood tests are negative. It is also for those who have never been given a diagnosis at all.

"When I first contacted Dr. Liebell, I had almost no short term memory left; even a brief 5 minute conversation with my husband was a challenge. I had to write myself notes so I could remember to do what was necessary to care for my preschool-aged son. I was often confused and could no longer follow text well enough to enjoy reading. I was in constant pain throughout my joints, muscles, and bones. The pain in my hands was so intense that I could no longer handle a full gallon of milk without assistance. I was completely unable to walk on my own. My husband carried me up and down the steps in our two-story home and I used a walker whenever I left our home. I blacked out while driving and totaled my car, and dizziness became a way of life. I struggled with migraines on a daily basis, often persisting for days or weeks at a time. I had both pneumonia and bronchitis multiple times. My vision worsened. I was always exhausted. I had heart palpitations that felt like my heart would stop for a second or two before picking back up again, usually accompanied by intense but brief chest pain. I also struggled with anxiety and panic attacks, to the point that my boss at the time had to call my husband to come pick me up because I was crying huddled in a corner.

The most upsetting thing for me personally was being told by my then-gynecologist that I would be unable to have biological children (my son is not my biological child), and that if I somehow managed to conceive a child, the baby would not make it to full term and I would most likely miscarry. I had a significant portion of my cervix surgically removed to get rid of some pre-cancerous growth that developed during this same time frame.

Besides seeing my regular family doctor, I saw a gynecologist, a cardiologist, an endocrinologist, and a neurologist. I was poked and prodded and examined to no avail. After thousands of dollars and countless medical appointments, I was only getting worse and no one could provide any answers. I was wrongly diagnosed with diabetes and had altered my diet considerably in an effort to improve my symptoms. I left my place of work as a pastry chef because my mind was so unclear and I needed to rest all the time. I didn't want to take long-term/lifelong antibiotics (plus our insurance wouldn't cover that treatment option anyway) so I was running out of options.

212

I was very cautious about both ear acupuncture and homeopathy, as neither was familiar to me. My husband thought it sounded like a hoax and I was tempted to agree before experiencing it firsthand. Needless to say, I went into my first appointment with Dr. Liebell carrying a heavy amount of skepticism with me… If he didn't so fully explain to me exactly what he was doing, I would not have even known tests were being done. He then placed a few very tiny needles in my outer ear and sealed them in place using a tiny square of tape. I could barely feel them go in, and I didn't feel them at all once they were actually in my ear… One of the needle's main functions for me was to provide some relief from my headaches. I was shocked to find that my migraines diminished significantly while the needle was in place! There was nothing scary or intimidating about any part of the process, and it was all very brief and painless. I especially appreciated the fact that Dr. Liebell constantly explained what he was doing and why it is was important.

I was given many homeopathic treatments to take at home. After racking up well over ten thousand dollars in medical bills from previous doctors that my health insurance wouldn't cover, this was a very welcome surprise. Honestly, I have spent less on health care with Dr. Liebell (including both the office visits and the homeopathic treatments) than I was spending just on co-pays previously. My husband noticed a difference in me before I did. After only a few weeks of treatment, my memory was beginning to improve significantly. I felt like I was in control of my own thoughts and once again was able to mentally participate in life! It was amazing.

All of my symptoms and medical problems have improved drastically. Some, like my short term memory, showed improvement after only a few weeks. Others took longer. After a little less than a year of treatment, I was able to walk well enough that I could abandon my walker and move on to a cane. After a couple of months with a cane, I am now walking and getting around completely on my own! I last used a cane in August 2012, right before my son's 6th birthday. After more than a year of not being able to walk on my own, this was the best feeling.

Shortly after I began to see Dr. Liebell, I found out I was pregnant! This was my first pregnancy and I was immediately panicked that my child would either get sick from my illness, or else get sick from my treatments. I contacted Dr. Liebell that same morning and spoke first with Barbara and then with the doctor. I was assured that not only were the treatments 100% safe during pregnancy, but that my continuation of the treatments would help prevent my baby from contracting any illness from me in utero. I remember crying on the phone because I was so scared for my baby (and in a state of shock since I was told we couldn't have children naturally). Both Barbara and Dr. Liebell were very comforting and gracious. My husband and I made the announcement to our families that same weekend! Throughout my pregnancy, during a time when most women become more and more uncomfortable, I was able to see my health improve dramatically. My pregnancy had no complications. And instead of being a high risk for miscarriage, my daughter actually carried past her due date by a week! I delivered my daughter Sadie on April 4, 2012 without painkillers or anesthesia. We brought her in to see Dr. Liebell, Barbara, and Sheila when she was a newborn. Sadie just celebrated her first birthday and to this day has not been sick once! She is the epitome of health.

Now that I am able to walk again, almost all of the pain in my body has disappeared. I rarely get a headache these days, and when I do it is mild by comparison. I am no longer anxious. I do still get dizzy sometimes but it is not a daily occurrence any more. My husband and I are also expecting another baby, due May 2013! I have regained so much strength also, especially in my hands and arms. Whereas I couldn't handle a full gallon of milk before, now I am able to carry around my one year old daughter for hours at a time and pick my 6 year old son up and spin him around. Such an amazing difference! Not only has my family grown by two since beginning treatment with Dr. Liebell, but I am able to be a better wife and mother to my family. I serve on the PTA board at my son's elementary school, I am actively involved in my church again instead of just being able to attend services, and I am able to participate in all of my family's activities and functions.

214

I cannot fully express how much my life has improved since I met Dr. Liebell. My husband would be quick to agree that his life has improved significantly as well. He can now come home and eat dinner and play with the kids and have a real conversation with his wife and finally enjoy his family again; no longer does he have to cook and clean and provide physical care to his wife and child after working a full day at his place of business with little or no rest.

Every time I have contact with anyone from the Liebell Clinic, it is a pleasant experience. The office at the Liebell Clinic is always clean and neat and peaceful. Whether interacting in person, over the phone, or via email, I am always regarded with kindness and respect. My children have accompanied me on visits as well as my father, and they are all always treated wonderfully as well. Depending on traffic, it takes us two to three hours each way for my appointments. The travel time isn't even a consideration because the care is so outstanding. The first time I called to inquire about the clinic and the treatment, my mind was in such a fog that I completely forgot why I had called in the first place. I was embarrassed and about to hang up the phone when Sheila quickly and reassuringly talked me through the situation by asking gentle questions. She told me that she had been there and she understood. (Imagine how I felt after months of no one understanding, and getting more than a few questioning glances from one-time friends, to have someone I didn't even know yet actually understand what I was experiencing! What a relief to not feel like I was losing my mind for once!) I made my first appointment and life has been gradually looking up ever since. My husband, my father, and I have told countless people about Dr. Liebell and the exemplary care I have received at the Liebell Clinic. I could not possibly give them a higher recommendation!

    - Tricia N., Chesterfield, Virginia 2013

"The doctor of the future will give no medicine but will interest his patients in the care of the human frame, in diet and in the cause and prevention of disease." - Thomas Edison

Chapter 26

The Weakest Link

Why Neck Health is a Critical Part of the Wellness Equation

Many sufferers of tick-triggered illness experience pain in the

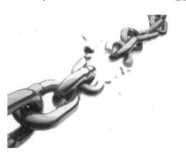

joints, tendons, muscles, and other related structures, and/or numbness or tingling in the hands or feet. Various frequently diagnosed nerve and arthritic disorders are common consequences, although scarcely correlated medically with tick-borne infection. For many, the temptation to blame every ache and pain on the effects of Lyme disease is irresistible. It is however, a dreadful mistake, which misdirects focus of treatment and causes needless suffering.

The great diversity of effects detonated by tick-borne infection stems from the tremendous physical differences of individual human bodies, and of equal significance, life experiences, conditions, and circumstances. One's history of injuries, personal stresses, genetic predispositions, and various other factors determine the course of tick-triggered illness and for that matter, health in general. Each person's unique weaknesses and strength are ultimately what determines the outcome.

For conditions such as acute Lyme disease, location and type of symptoms may be determined by what tissues are most susceptible in each individual. For example, a person might have a history of neck problems initially precipitated by an auto accident many years prior to an infectious tick bite. That person's neck may permanently remain the "weak link," leaving it the focus of symptoms generated by new irritants in the form of *Borrelia* and other microbes. For other people, the fingers, the knees, the gastrointestinal system, or the brain might be the weakened areas—the easy targets.

Primary vs. Secondary Conditions

Over 2,000 years ago, Socrates said we live in a world of law governed by a system of order, whether we understand the principles behind it or not. He taught people to think logically about the consequences of their thoughts and behaviors. Everybody knows this today as the *Law of Cause and Effect.* It simply means that everything happens for a reason. There is a cause, or a series of specific, measurable causes that might be identified. We accept this scientifically-proven fact today, but in Socrates' day it was a controversial idea, which was one of the reasons he was put to death! Of course, Sir Isaac Newton eventually proved it in physics—that every action has an equal and opposite reaction.

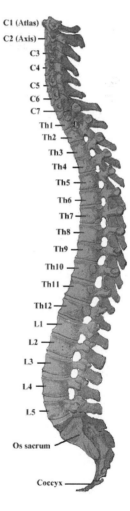

217

A primary condition is one for which the symptoms are the *direct* result of its cause or causes. Secondary conditions are more chronic developments activated as a result of a primary underlying cause. However, the signs and symptoms are not caused *directly* by the primary problem, but rather due to a domino effect. As I described earlier in the chapter on diagnosis, a great many common medical conditions are secondary conditions, for which the primary cause may never be even considered, let alone adequately treated. Diagnoses such as migraines, peripheral neuropathy, fibromyalgia, or multiple sclerosis are all examples of secondary conditions for which medications are typically prescribed to suppress and manage symptoms. Their *primary* causes may be any combination of infection, toxicity, structural problems, genetics, and personal stresses and circumstances. I am certain that one of the major reasons so many people suffer complex chronic pain and illness is treating the symptoms of secondary problems, and ignoring their primary causes.

Medically confirmed tick-borne infection is a legitimate *primary* condition which is clearly capable of triggering a cascade of different *secondary* problems which apparently can persist and progress long after active infection has been competently cleared. Their diagnoses may indeed be legitimately accurate by medical standards, but they do not account for the primary causes. But this is undoubtedly not always the case. Lyme *Borrelia* or any other infection may also function as a secondary condition that *exacerbates* or magnifies multiple existing health conditions. This appears to be the case even after antibiotic treatment appears to have successfully cleared active infection. Perhaps this is the truth behind many cases designated as chronic Lyme disease, or post-treatment Lyme disease syndrome. Viewing Lyme disease through this lens makes it clear that its symptoms may be either primary or secondary conditions.

218

Throughout this book, I have expressed my distaste for classifying Lyme disease as a "mimic" or "great imitator" of other medical conditions. Lyme is better branded as a great *instigator*. However, Lyme is hardly unique in this regard. Countless types of microorganisms can equally spark the development of disease. The same holds true for chemical toxins, as well as *structural problems*.

> **"Get knowledge of the spine,**
> **for this is the requisite for many diseases."**
> – Hippocrates, the Father of Modern Medicine
> (460-370 BC), Corpus Hippocrateum

The axiom, a chain is only as strong as its weakest link is highly relevant. The spine is without a doubt, a part of the body that needs considerable attention, and can often be the "weak link in the chain." Any area of the body that has been previously stressed, damaged, or diseased may maintain lowered tissue resistance. This means it is more susceptible to any stress than stronger and healthier body structures or systems. Lyme infection is but one such potential hazard in an infinite sea of microbes and other substances that may infiltrate the human body.

Thus far, I have discussed the importance of clearing energetic blockages to healing by means of auricular therapy and the homeopathic effect. However, detection and correction of *structural* blockages must be considered too. A bio-*mechanical* problem in the spine can cause a bio-*energetic* disturbance: interference to conduction of nerve signal transmission. Nerves are just like wires that send electrical signals to tell the body what to do. The nervous system is the body's master system. The spine, which houses and protects the spinal cord is like the circuit breaker box for the entire body.

Self-Healing vs. Self-Correcting

Ultimately, it is still *energy* that breathes life into physical structures, in a similar manner to how electricity powers machines. The difference is that living bodies are *not* machines. A machine cannot heal itself by regenerating and repairing its own physical parts. The human body does so in an awe-inspiring manner—provided nothing *blocks* the natural process. The human body is self-healing—but it is not always self-*correcting*. There's a big difference between the two. Broken bones and dislocations are obvious and extreme examples. For example, in 1990, I suffered a severe dislocation of my middle finger joint from falling on the ice in my driveway in New York. Had the doctor at the hospital not swiftly and competently set the bone back in alignment, it would have healed permanently and painfully 45 degrees crooked. It was critical for a highly-skilled doctor to correct the structural problem so my finger would be able to heal itself functionally.

The human spine at times, cannot correct itself from mechanical problems. It is a magnificent and complex structure composed of individual bones (vertebrae), which interlock to form joints. These joints function together as one cohesive synchronized unit. Each individual bone/joint needs to move properly, and has a normal range of motion. However, the joints of the spine can get stuck—like rusty hinges. There are circumstances where the muscles cannot physically unlock them. This can result in various consequences, including local inflammation, nerve interference, and abnormal mechanics of other joints of the body. This in turn, can cause many medical problems, which are given different names (secondary diagnoses). Neck and back pain barely scratch the surface of what can go wrong. When spinal joints are stuck—they must be physically corrected so the body can heal itself. This is not a *muscle* problem for which physical therapy, exercises, or massage would be effective.

220

The human body can indeed heal itself from many problems when mechanical and neurological blockages are reduced. Manual treatment of the spine dates back to ancient Greece, Egypt, China, Native America, and elsewhere. Doctors of chiropractic have long been the experts specifically trained to address this aspect of human health. Treatment is accomplished through various hand or instrument-delivered techniques. It is referred to as chiropractic *adjustment*.

> ## "Look to the nervous system as the key to maximum health."
> - Claudius Galen (130-202 AD) "Prince of Physicians"

Electrochemical signals are transmitted from the brain, down the spinal cord, and out through openings in the spine to the entire body. These nerve impulses return to the brain via the same route. Proper nerve signal transmission is essential to the function of all organs and tissues. Anything that interferes with this process creates a blockage to normal function, and thus can impair healing. Consider a machine's electrical system being compromised by a faulty mechanical system. If the wires cannot properly conduct electricity because a mechanical problem is interfering with the wires— the machine will not function properly. Nerves are the human "wires," which if interfered with, can result in various symptoms and illness.

Chiropractic treatment (adjustments) are not for bones... they are for *nerves*! This has always been the case since the profession's formal introduction in 1895 (Davenport, Iowa). A doctor of chiropractic adjusts the spine to clear the structural

221

blockage to nerve impulse transmission. The chiropractic terminology for abnormal spinal mechanics that are causing nerve interference is *vertebral subluxation.*

Doctors of Chiropractic (D.C.) are primary health care providers licensed in all 50 U.S. states. Chiropractic is extremely safe and highly effective to support natural healing of many problems. Obviously the benefits of chiropractic treatment are scientifically acknowledged, since these methods are covered by federal government-contracted health insurance policies (Medicare, Blue Cross/Blue Shield, Mail handlers).

It is sad-but-true that the majority of conventional medical doctors still seldom prescribe chiropractic care instead of, or in addition to drugs and surgery. Like homeopathy, chiropractic was not *invented* by members of the *American Medical Association* (AMA). It does not fit into their lucrative business model of drug and surgery-based health care. In 1987, a U.S. Federal court found the AMA guilty of conspiracy to destroy the chiropractic profession!

My family and the patients I have treated since 1992, are grateful for chiropractic, homeopathy, and acupuncture—three magnificent holistic healing arts which the AMA has ruthlessly tried to destroy. Despite chiropractic's impeccable track record for safety and effectiveness, it has been treated as a threat to the financial interests of the pharmaceutical and surgery industry. Many great books and articles have been written exposing this and other dastardly indiscretions and the cutthroat business tactics of mainstream medicine, so I will not elaborate further.

In a more civilized and caring medical system, chiropractic would be considered as an effective and necessary treatment option—part of the complete "tool box" of health care. There's a time and a place for all kinds of medical treatment. No one type of doctor is qualified to do everything. It is foolish to seek out a general physician for dental problems. Dentists are the teeth experts. A cardiologist would be the wrong doctor to call upon for *eye* problems. A chiropractor would be the wrong choice for heart surgery, but should be the first choice for non-surgical spine-related problems. No other type of doctor studies about, and attends to the spine like a chiropractor. All health care professionals should at least be *aware* of the various specialties and treatment options for their patients. Like homeopathy, bio-energetic supplementation, auricular therapy, and traditional acupuncture, chiropractic is not a direct treatment for any disease in the conventional medical sense. Doctors of chiropractic have been the American pioneers and leaders of the holistic health movement since 1895. We have *always* been the advocates of treating the body as a whole—emphasizing diet, exercise, and prevention, in addition to maintaining spinal health. Today, we see various conventional medical doctors proclaiming these principles as if they were *new* ideas.

Tick Infection and Neck Inspection

It is an undisputed scientific fact that spinal problems can have far-reaching health consequences. Many symptoms exist because of mechanical and neurological problems in the spine—**the upper neck,** in particular. Tick-borne infection may indeed intensify the effects of such, even if not the primary cause. I have consistently found that tiny imbalances in the upper neck are responsible for many of the neurological, joint, and muscular symptoms for which Lyme disease had inaccurately been implicated as the sole cause. In my experience, those who are afflicted by chronic tick-triggered illness respond better when expertly-administered chiropractic treatment is part of the equation—with particular emphasis on the upper neck.

223

The greatest concentration of nerve connections in the human body is at the junction where the brain extends out through the base of skull, continuing down as the brain stem and spinal cord. The medical term for this region is the **upper cervical spine**, which includes the top two bones of the neck called the **atlas and axis vertebrae**. These two vertebrae look completely different from those in the rest of the spine. The atlas is a two-ounce bone that supports the weight of the skull (averaging between 9-17 pounds!). The atlas vertebra is often referred to as C1. "C" stands for cervical spine, which simply means neck.

Are YOU Carrying the Weight of the World on Your Shoulders?

Why is the first bone of the neck called Atlas? In Greek mythology the titan, Atlas was responsible for bearing the weight of the heavens on his shoulders, a burden given to him as punishment by Zeus. Consider holding up a bowling ball with a Dixie cup. That is similar to the tremendous physical responsibility and burden of the atlas vertebra. The C2 vertebra—the second bone of the neck is called the **axis**. It forms the axis of rotation for the atlas in the form of a pivot joint. The first 45 degrees of head rotation takes place here before the rest of the joints of the neck kick in.

What Goes Wrong with the Upper Neck?

Upper Cervical Stenosis (UCS) is an extremely common problem that is rarely considered by mainstream medicine. Unless one has a fracture, dislocation, gross deformity, or abnormal growth, the upper cervical spine is rarely given a thought. However, it has been verified that a nearly imperceptible narrowing of the spinal canal caused by mechanical imbalance between the top two vertebrae and the skull, can silently "choke" the spinal cord—leading to nerve interference, which can potentially affect any area of the body. It may be present as early as at birth, but various painful symptoms may take years, or even decades to develop before nerve compression becomes severe enough, due to age-related spinal degeneration or specifically, spinal trauma. Like Lyme disease, UCS can be the primary cause of many symptoms for which people receive a wide variety of secondary diagnoses. Nerve interference at the base of one's skull can produce many of the symptoms erroneously assumed to be due to Lyme disease! UCS can exist at the same time as Lyme, creating a devastating one-two punch. In my clinical experience, many people develop neurological, joint, and muscular symptoms because their already existing spinal problems become severely magnified as the result of tick-borne infection and/or its post-treatment residual effects.

From the moment we are born, our spines are often traumatized. The birth process itself can harm a baby's neck, although commonly unnoticed. Even in a normal birth, it can be subjected to significant twisting and pulling forces that have significant consequences. Research from Germany in 1987 revealed that babies suffered a wide range of health problems due to blocked nerve impulses caused by correctable misalignment of the upper neck. Cited in the study were cases of lowered resistance to infection!

(Source: Gutman G: *"Blocked atlantal nerve syndrome in infants and small children."* published in *"Manuelle Medizin,"* Springer-Verlag, 1987. Published in English, *International Review of Chiropractic* 1990 46(4):37)

> **"If you would seek health,
> look first to the spine."**
> - Socrates (469-399 BC)

An old neck injury can be a hidden primary condition that can be worsened by tick-borne infection. A study published in the *Journal of Whiplash and Related Disorders* reported that neck injuries commonly cause significant problems, long-term complications, and disabilities which are largely unresponsive to treatment from many medical disciplines. For example, many auto accident victims eventually develop symptoms ultimately diagnosed as fibromyalgia. They are doomed and destined to a lifetime of prescription medications to manage the symptoms that were caused by shamefully unconsidered and untreated upper neck injury. Millions of Americans have been diagnosed with fibromyalgia. It is a fantastic example of a secondary condition. "Authorities" say its causes are either unknown or unclear. I beg to differ!

The *University of Kansas School of Medicine and Arthritis Research Center* studied the relationship between neck injury and fibromyalgia. The conclusion of this study (161 cases) revealed that fibromyalgia was 13 times more frequent following neck injury, compared to other areas of the body! Many of these patients had no characteristic symptoms prior to some sort of neck trauma, which may have taken place many years prior to the onset of the mysterious symptoms labeled fibromyalgia. Even though not all fibromyalgia patients remember having a specific neck injury, imbalances of the upper cervical spine are routinely found.

Fibromyalgia is a diagnosis very familiar to many victims of tick-triggered illness. In my clinical experience, upper cervical stenosis and tick-borne infection (or past history of it) are the two most important considerations for those afflicted with symptoms associated with fibromyalgia. Many people are victims of tick-borne infection regardless of noticing a tick and/or its allegedly classic associated rash. Equally, many people are completely unaware of any injury or strain to the upper neck, or they simply do not remember such an

226

occurrence. Both of these extremely common problems are virtually ignored medically. It is appalling that evaluation for the subtle-but-serious effects of upper cervical stenosis is not a vital part of routine health evaluation. It is a frighteningly illogical omission. Neglecting to consider one of the most significant neurological regions of the body is unconscionable. Yet, most people only receive spinal treatment later in life, once there is significant pain or visible degeneration. Even worse, treatment for neck problems comes mostly in the form of arthritis drugs, futile exercises, and surgery. Fortunately, there is a solution…

Upper Cervical Care

Upper cervical chiropractors are the only doctors licensed, trained, and qualified in the specific, non-surgical treatment of the atlas and axis vertebrae. They receive additional certification beyond the general licensure of doctor of chiropractic (D.C.), through accredited and recognized professional institutions. Medical doctors (MD) are not qualified unless they also have additionally earned a doctoral degree in chiropractic, plus upper cervical certification. There are several different outstanding upper cervical techniques practiced around the world. They are all outstanding, and I wholeheartedly endorse any of them.

Upper cervical care has been my area of specialty since 1992, with an emphasis on helping people diagnosed by other physicians with fibromyalgia. I have proudly helped people with many unresolved chronic ailments by focusing on the upper neck with an extraordinary procedure called **Atlas Orthogonal**. It was introduced in 1970 by the ingenious Dr. Roy W. Sweat of Atlanta, Georgia. What a privilege and an honor I have had to have been trained by him, and board certified through his program. Atlas Orthogonal is a marvel of science, technology, skill, experience, and love. It is a cutting-edge, mathematically-based, rehabilitative treatment performed with a safe and delicate sound wave instrument. Each person's treatment is as unique as a fingerprint. A sophisticated mathematical x-ray analysis is performed to determine each individual's specific treatment. In mathematics, orthogonal refers to the relation of two lines at right angles to one another (perpendicular)

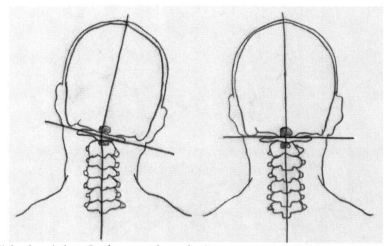

With the Atlas Orthogonal analysis, we are measuring (to a fraction of a degree) the position of the skull in relation to the atlas vertebra and the rest of the neck. The mathematical analysis enables the doctor to precisely adjust the atlas vertebra back towards normal (orthogonal) position. The measurements and calculations are like finding a specific combination to a lock. The "lock" is your upper neck! The Atlas Orthogonal procedure re-aligns the bones of the upper neck with the skull. This reduces the stenosis (narrowing) of the spinal canal. This in turn, reduces the pressure on the spinal cord/brain stem region, the meninges, as well as blood vessels, to restore normal function. Treating structural problems of the upper neck with Atlas Orthogonal improves nerve function. This can directly result in elimination of pain. It is not a "quick fix," but rather a rehabilitative regimen. Nevertheless, results are often rapid and dramatic. This completely painless procedure has unparalleled safety.

In the whiplash study mentioned earlier, Atlas Orthogonal was put to the test—with extraordinary results. It was revealed to be highly effective for chronic pain sufferers for whom multiple conventional medical treatments had previously failed. It was quite a big deal for a study on a chiropractic procedure to be published in a mainstream medical journal. I am proud to be among the relatively few doctors in the world who specialize in this astonishing non-surgical corrective treatment for the upper cervical spine. It is without a doubt the most underutilized procedure and best-kept secret in all of health care. This is why my original website is called necksecret.com!

"One of the worst problems was the pain in my neck. A surgeon told me to take hot showers, and that I had arthritis and nothing could be done. That was 9 years ago... A sports doctor put me on Paxil and I was taking Voltarin for "arthritis." He sent me to physical therapy, but it never took the pain away. By the second week of treatment [with Atlas Orthogonal] I was flying high—I felt wonderful. I guess for the last 4 or 5 years, I didn't know what it was like to sleep the whole night through."
- Joyce W., Virginia Beach, 2000

Is it in the Genes?

While our genes play a role in the development of health problems, our environment and circumstances weigh in heavily. The *sickness* philosophy of health care teaches that genes are our destiny. This is patently untrue. If our destinies were purely determined by genes, we would consistently suffer all of the same ailments of our ancestors, and we would not live long. Our genes are but one component of our health destiny. Being vulnerable, susceptible or having a genetic predisposition (the medical term) for illness does not make any illness an inevitable outcome. You learned earlier (in the chapter on energy fields) that genes are *not* the fundamental "blueprints" of our bodies. Electric fields influence the DNA. Our genes do not fully explain the tremendous capabilities of our bodies.

Lyme Disease, Multiple Sclerosis
and the Upper Cervical Spine...
Is There a Connection?

Published academic medical literature has indicated a connection between Lyme disease and multiple sclerosis. Like anything to do with Lyme disease, it sparks controversy. As I state throughout this book, with my holistic wellness approach, I steer clear of such nonsense. Whether or not MS is caused by *Borrelia* infection is immaterial. Any admission of such within the scientific community would inevitably end up politicized in debate over antibiotics, insurance coverage, and money. My suspicion is that those afflicted by MS have some degree of genetic weakness for which an infectious tick bite might trigger the autoimmune response that causes the characteristic nerve damage of the disease. Another person bitten by the same tick might struggle with only arthritis in the knees, or perhaps headaches...or nothing!

Like Lyme infection, upper neck dysfunction has also been implicated with multiple sclerosis. On December 18, 2008 Emmy Award-winning talk show host Montel Williams publicly endorsed upper cervical chiropractic on his program. In 1999, he was diagnosed with multiple sclerosis, and suffered severe and constant daily nerve pain in the legs, as well as balance problems. Montel then visited my colleague, Dr. Patrick Kerr. Dr. Kerr is board certified in the Atlas Orthogonal upper cervical chiropractic method, as am I. The improvements Montel experienced were astonishing. He told his audience that he was already walking better, had regained leg strength, and decreased pain. He added that he was able to stand up straight without pain for the first time in over five years! Montel Williams proclaimed his experience with Atlas Orthogonal, *"the most amazing thing that has ever happened to me"*

The video of the segment can be seen at:
http://www.liebellclinic.com/atlas-orthogonal.html

The connection between the neck and multiple sclerosis goes well beyond Montel's experience. A preliminary research study published in the *Journal of Vertebral Subluxation Research* established that neck trauma can be a factor in the development of MS, as well as Parkinson's disease. The 81-patient study revealed that upper cervical chiropractic corrections could enable improvements for both conditions.

(Source: *Eighty-One Patients with Multiple Sclerosis and Parkinson's Disease Undergoing Upper Cervical Chiropractic Care to Correct Vertebral Subluxation: A Retrospective Analysis.* J. Vertebral Subluxation Res. - JVSR.Com, August 2, 2004. Erin L. Elster, D.C.)

The Upper Neck and Chronic Headaches

Many victims of Lyme disease and other tick-borne infection blame their chronic headaches solely on infection. While this can certainly be the case, dysfunction of the upper cervical spine is an extremely common cause, which must always be considered. Yet it rarely *is* medically, despite the publicized conclusions of several highly-respected researchers. Nikolai Bogduk, MD, PhD, has served as Professor of Anatomy at the university in Newcastle, Australia. He is a world-renowned research scientist, who supports the neck-based approach to headaches. He has expressed his outrage that those in control of the headache treatment field will not recognize or act upon the knowledge that the neck-based model of headaches is the best evolved one for a high percentage of headaches. Years ago, another medical researcher and anesthesiologist, Peter Rothbart, M.D., came to the same conclusion, declaring in the Toronto Star newspaper that doctors of chiropractic had been correct all along regarding headaches.

The medical term for neck-related headaches is *cervicogenic headache*. My observation has been that this term, as well as any published medical research that has proven the anatomical relation between headaches and the neck, has been ignored. I have recently been hearing the term, occipital neuralgia. This refers to irritation to nerves residing at the upper neck/skull region. I have had patients report to me that they were diagnosed as such by neurologists and other specialists. My gut feeling is that the name was changed by the mainstream medical establishment from cervicogenic headache to occipital neuralgia to prevent doctors of chiropractic from the opportunity to help millions of headache suffers get well. Regardless of the name given to such headaches, I am certain that chiropractic specialists in upper cervical spine are eminently qualified to be the leaders in the field of correcting the cause of chronic headaches for millions of people worldwide.

"For many years my neck bothered me almost every morning. When I'd look up, tilting my head back, my hearing would mysteriously cut out. I also had headaches every single day. As a professional ballet instructor, I was unable to demonstrate properly because of the pain... Now, thanks to Dr. Liebell and Atlas correction, I'm finally out of pain. My life is so much better. I sleep better than ever. Now I know how important your nervous system and spinal alignment is. My hearing problem is gone too, as a result of atlas corrections! Now I can get up in the morning without neck pain, and I rarely get headaches! - Michael K., Norfolk, Virginia

Your Atlas Vertebra and Your Immune System

Nicholas Gonzalez, M.D. was a well-known, New York-based immunologist and cancer specialist. He appeared on many television and radio programs to discuss his patients' remarkable successes with intensive enzyme and nutritional therapy alternatives for cancer. Dr. Gonzalez revealed that the majority of his patients also have obvious neck problems, even without

232

recollection of any trauma. I met Dr. Gonzalez many years ago at an Atlas Orthogonal seminar for which he spoke. He was a brilliant man with a heart of gold, who like all of us unconventional doctors had to fight hard for the opportunity to help suffering people, who want effective health care beyond the mere prescription of drugs. Dr. Gonzalez was an ardent advocate of the Atlas Orthogonal procedure. He expressed his sadness over how millions of people could be helped by it, but do not know it exists. His stance was that if neck function is faulty—nutrition will not be assimilated properly. Nerve function can interfere with immune function and reduce chances of recovery.

> *"90% of the stimulation and nutrition to the brain is generated by the movement of the spine"*
> **- Dr. Roger Sperry, (Nobel Prize Recipient for Brain Research)**
> 1988, Bulletin of Theosophy Science Study Group 26(3-4), 27-28.
> Nerve Connections. Quarterly Review Biology. 46, 198.

While there is certainly a greater need for further academic scientific research to be published, my patients and I agree precision upper neck correction supports immune function via improved nerve function. This is why it is part of the *Bio-energetic Individual Treatment Equation.* Our goal is to improve spinal health and function, utilizing highly-specialized and structured chiropractic approaches, which can be reproduced with consistent results from patient to patient.

Chiropractic Resources:

I am certain everybody should have chiropractic spinal treatment. However, I do not personally endorse any specific doctors listed through any of the below resources. They list doctors specializing in upper neck-focused methods, including myself. What is ultimately the most important thing is that you get the best chiropractor you can find, regardless of any specific technique. My best recommendation is to get a referral from somebody you know and trust for a great doctor of chiropractic close to your home or workplace.

www.upcspine.com
(Patient advocate-created international website with largest international directory of upper cervical specialists)

www.uppercervicalsubluxation.com
(Journal of Upper Cervical Research)

www.uppercervical.org
(Patient Advocate Created Website)

www.necksecret.com
(The Liebell Clinic website)

www.globalao.com
(Official Website of Atlas Orthogonal method)

www.uppercervicalcare.com
(Upper Cervical Centers of America)

www.blairchiropractic.com
(Official Website of Blair Method)

www.orthospinology.org
(Official Website of Orthospinology Method)

www.nucca.org
(Official Website of NUCCA method)

Chapter 27

Vitamin D Deficiency Dilemma

Vitamin D is critical for the function of muscles, joints, sleep cycle, your moods, and numerous other aspects of a healthy body. If you are low in vitamin D, your body doesn't use calcium properly, or absorb it from your diet. Some of the muscle aches attributed to Lyme disease are due to low vitamin D levels and regulation. Scientific studies have proven that vitamin D is a significant factor towards natural improvement from many health problems.

Vitamin D is more accurately classified as a hormone rather than a nutrient. Technically vitamins are carbon-based compounds that your body needs for normal function that it cannot manufacture on its own. Hormones, on the other hand are more complex compounds that are produced by the *body* itself for various functions. There are only a few dietary sources of vitamin D. If your level is low, it would be very difficult, unlikely, inconvenient, and expensive to restore it to normal through diet. Every day, you would have to eat ridiculously large quantities of salmon, sardines, and egg yolks, which would be not be healthful, desirable or feasible.

In a perfect world, everybody would produce vitamin D in the skin via sunlight exposure. When ultraviolet B rays of sunlight (UVB) hit your skin, it triggers your body to produce a substance called **cholecalciferol**. This gets converted by your liver into **calcidiol**. Then, through addition of an enzyme, the kidneys convert it to **calcitriol**, which is the active form of vitamin D.

According to world renowned cancer specialist (oncologist) Yoshiaki Omura, MD, ultraviolet radiation from the sun has increased to the point that it has become very difficult to safely generate adequate vitamin D3 production via skin exposure. He has concluded that the cancer risks are greater than the benefit. Thus, determining the most effective dosages of vitamin D supplementation for each individual is essential. According to Dr. Omura's published medical research, expertly-determined optimum daily supplemental dosage of vitamin D3 is tremendously supportive to patients with numerous serious health conditions (especially cancer).

Dr. Omura is a research scientist, a humanitarian, and a bonafide genius. His remarkable background in both Western and Eastern medicine has given him unparalleled scientific qualifications. Dr. Omura has one of the most impressive medical resumes one could imagine. He is an oncologist, cardiologist, surgeon, acupuncturist, electro-physicist, and medical school professor. However, his primary methods are natural treatments and non-invasive diagnostic methods. **Most of Dr. Omura's patients' success is attributable to his method of determining each patient's optimal daily dose of vitamin D3.** This might not seem like a big deal on the surface. However, it is of *monumental* importance. How it is done is the key! Although many people are *already* taking vitamin D supplements, Dr. Omura has found that commonly-recommended dosages (and frequency of usage) are ineffective and potentially harmful. This can make or break a person's chance to overcome many illnesses.

Dr. Yoshiaki Omura has published over 270 original research articles, many chapters, and 9 books. At age 84, he is currently

(2018) Adjunct Professor of Family & Community Medicine, NY Medical College. Dr. Omura is the President and Professor of the International College of Acupuncture and Electro-Therapeutics, NY, as well as the Editor in Chief, Acupuncture & Electro-Therapeutics Research, International Journal of Integrative Medicine. I have studied his wealth of medical research papers, and have had the privilege to observe him evaluating and advising cancer patients in New York City.

In my practice, I exclusively implement Dr. Omura's methods for vitamin D supplementation: Bi-digital O-ring Testing (BDORT), discussed in Chapter 21. **Dr. Omura and I agree that most multivitamins (and many other vitamin supplements) are potentially harmful, and should usually be avoided. They are concentrated mixtures of substances that do not go together well.** Dr. Omura has tested them for decades. There are indeed supplements that *alone* may be beneficial; however, they can commonly be harmful when combined with others. We must determine this for each individual using BDORT.

Let me be crystal clear that I am not claiming vitamin D3 as a cure for any disease. However, a significant amount of medical research suggests its importance in support of many ailments. Using Dr. Omura's patented, inexpensive, non-invasive method (BDORT), I determine each person's daily optimal vitamin D3 dosage (taken every 7-8 hours). We use a very inexpensive brand of vitamin D3 supplement tablets, chosen as the result of Dr. Omura's years of research testing products from countless manufacturers. In most cases, the optimal daily dosage is drastically less than the commonly-recommended 50,000 international units per week. This is an important part of the wellness-promoting equation. Those who suffer the chronic effects of tick-triggered illness notoriously have vitamin D problems, yet have not responded well to past supplementation (even with large long-term dosages).

"Shall I refuse my dinner because I do not fully understand the process of digestion?" - Oliver Heaviside (1850-1925) English physicist.

Chapter 28

Fantastic Food Fortification

Why Superior Nutrition Obtained Through Whole Foods Beats Taking Expensive, Processed Vitamin and Mineral Supplements

Perhaps you've been told vegetables don't have the nutrient content like they used to due to depletion of nutrients in the soil. Vitamin manufacturers certainly insist a regular diet doesn't contain enough vitamins. Assuming this is true, it is still not a sound argument for haphazardly consuming mega-doses of processed supplements. Rather it is motivation to make better food choices and consumption. There is evidence that taking too many of some vitamins and minerals (including calcium and iron) can cause harm. They can even cause drug interactions (note: bio-energetic supplements and homeopathy do NOT). **Supplements have risks.** For example, a German and Swiss research report suggested that calcium supplements can significantly increase heart attack risk compared to fairly high intake of calcium rich *foods,* such as green leafy vegetables, sardines, sesame seeds, and dairy. According to *Consumer Reports,* between 2007 and 2012, the FDA received more than 6,300 reports of serious adverse events linked to dietary supplements, including vitamins and herbs. It included 115 deaths, more than 2,100 hospitalizations, and several thousand other medical complications.

Stay Safe: Get Nutrients from Food—Not Pills

Our bodies can extract nutrients from food, at the right speed, and at the right amounts. Sudden bombardment of some nutrients can be overwhelming and STRESSFUL to your body. **Most vitamin pills have ingredients that are far from natural.** They are legally permitted by the FDA. By law, vitamins don't have to come from nature! It's enough that government regulated and tested *drugs* are one of the leading causes of death in America. Let's not assume that supplements are the harmless health miracle they're portrayed to be. According to world-renowned cancer specialist, Yoshiaki Omura, MD, without individually examining chemical interaction, we cannot safely combine supplements. Many have drug interactions which can reduce or cancel effectiveness of other treatments. Individual testing is absolutely critical. This is why I use bio-energetic testing methods to evaluate individual needs.

When human beings stop eating whole foods, it becomes necessary to delve into the complexities of biochemistry. However, if we eat a wide variety of whole foods in a truly natural manner, we do not really have to much at all about vitamins, minerals, enzymes, trace elements, and other substances that are the objects of study in the field of clinical nutrition. With the *Bio-energetic Individual Treatment Equation*© the broccoli, the organic chicken and eggs, the blueberries, raw seeds and nuts, and dozens of other inherently nutritious *real* foods automatically possess the "knowledge" of nutrition. If we eat lots of whole foods it is not necessary to have a doctoral degree in nutrition. Keep in mind that diet is not the answer to everything either. I suggest nutrition through whole natural foods rather than pills. You've got to spend money on food— so why buy loads of supplements too… just spend a bit more on higher quality food. And I highly recommend you check out my "Quick Health Advice" page on my website:

https://www.chronic-lyme-disease-solutions.com/general-health-advice.html

Organic or Not, Here I Come

I am an ardent advocate of whole food nutrition, exercise, fresh air, sunshine, and all that is good and natural. Nevertheless, it has not been *these* things that have propelled my patients back to a state of health. Many a consumer of the finest organic produce and grass-fed meats has presented to me in the same sorry state of tick-triggered illness as those who eat fast food and haven't eaten a vegetable in decades!

I applaud authors who provide dietary advice and recipes for sufferers of Lyme disease. I solidly support any measures that may reduce inflammation in the body. Eating more whole foods that are free of harmful processed ingredients is great general health advice. However, I consistently see patients for whom strict dietary changes, as well as massive dosages of nutritional supplements have not made the slightest dent in their illness! I always encourage improving healthy lifestyle habits, but diet simply has not been my patients' key to success. I have been privileged and thrilled to witness the recovery of people who eat mediocre or fairly poor diets *equally* to those living extremely health-oriented lifestyles. This is of course, not as an endorsement for you to subsist upon fast food, soda, cigarettes, and beer.

We never know what deck of cards we are each dealt genetically. Each person has different strengths and weaknesses. I have no doubt that every patient's best chances for success include good nutrition. The problem there is what constitutes the best nutrition for each person differs. In most cases, I have found it *stressful* for patients to suddenly change dietary habits. With few exceptions, I find (using bio-energetic testing methods) most supplemental pills, capsules, and liquids to be excessive in recommended dosages, and frequently detrimental to progress. I am certain natural healing is best supported by natural foods.

240

Chapter 29

Navigating the Road to Wellness

The pain relief medicine industry flourishes because the public has been well-trained (dare I say, brainwashed) to seek drugs to make them feel better—regardless of the consequences towards their health. I'm hardly unsympathetic when it comes to pain (my office door does say Chronic Pain Solutions!). However, it is my experience that progressive and lasting improvement sometimes requires weathering the storm of a healing crisis. Within 1-3 weeks of beginning a regimen of bio-energetic supplementation, approximately forty percent of patients experience a natural exacerbation of existing symptoms, or reoccurrence of old symptoms. This is referred to as a **healing crisis.** It may last a day, or occasionally, a week or so.

It is indeed a lot easier to numb the pain rather than correct the causes, and rehabilitate and repair long-term damage and dysfunction. Many elite professional athletes have had to go through extremely difficult and painful rehabilitation from injuries. Clearly, it's not always as simple as taking a pill or getting a shot. For some patients, the road to recovery is difficult—no pain, no gain, as the cliché aptly goes. Everybody wants to feel better as quickly as possible. We should indeed be grateful for the existence of prescription medications that provide relief. Natural methods sometimes just don't cut the mustard. However, one of the great tragedies of Western medical philosophy is trading long-term improvement and resolution of illness for instant gratification. Persistently pandering to pain with symptom-masking drugs merely delivers the illusion of health. It does nothing to drive you towards wellness. Health is much more than simply the absence of symptoms. It is well-known that some of the most serious illnesses, such as cancer and heart disease do not present with symptoms until they've gotten really bad.

Think about it: an overweight, physically unfit, and chronically ill person cannot (under any circumstances) be given a pill or any other type of treatment, and radically transform into a slim, athletic and strong, and healthy individual overnight. Yet that is what has become *expected* from medical care—because that is what marketers of medicine, fitness gadgets, and weight loss pills have been promising. By contrast, with the BITE, no such outlandish and unrealistic promises are made, nor are they expected. We do however, have high expectations, accompanied by realistic time frames. Getting better from complex, chronic, and degenerative illnesses takes time. The road to recovery has challenges. It has its ups and downs. When your body is gradually and naturally eliminating long-accumulated toxins, and overcoming chronic infection, it can be unpleasant.

Smooth Sailing and Setbacks

The black dashed line on the next page's graph hypothetically depicts progress as a steady improvement over time—the patient feeling a little better each day. This however, is not reality—for most things in life! The solid line is what we expect: various ups and downs while climbing the mountain toward the goal of wellness. Notice that even though there are improvements and setbacks represented by the jagged red graph line—the trend is still upwards. This is the true-to-life progression of the natural road to wellness.

242

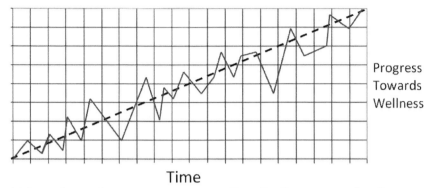

Progress
Towards
Wellness

Time

Although we do see some extraordinarily fast recoveries from chronic pain and illness, getting better naturally is usually a slow and gradual, but rewarding process. Be mindful that it is also not necessarily smooth sailing from start to finish. While progressing toward wellness, you can be doing great for a while, but still have setbacks. The catchphrase, "two steps forward, one step back," is applicable. Additionally, it is helpful to adopt the philosophy that slow progress beats no progress!

It's important to know this in advance, so you don't have unrealistic expectations. This means that you will not necessarily simply feel better and better with time and effort. Life has many stresses, including physical challenges, and exposures to *new* illnesses. One can experience colds, flu, and other infections, as well as suffering injuries, and fatigue while progressing on the journey toward recovery from existing *chronic* illness. Every symptom you experience while on your wellness journey is not a direct response to treatment, nor are all symptoms related to your chronic problems. Be mindful that we are exposed regularly to viruses, bacteria, fungi, and a host of other parasites in our air, food, and through contact with others. There are chemical toxins everywhere, as well as radiation from technology. Emotional stress plays an equally important role.

One may have twenty or more different chronic problems from various causes—some related to each other, and some not. As one problem gets better, others can become more noticeable. You could have five of the twenty original problems get completely better, but you're still left with fifteen other things that are making you miserable. That's where another great cliché becomes pertinent: patience is a virtue! Progressive improvement from chronic illness can require toughing it out, and getting through an initial stage of healing, which may not feel good.

Healing Crisis vs. Herxheimer Reaction — What is the Difference?

It appears clinically that the information imprints embedded within the solutions of the bio-energetic supports give your body a heightened awareness of its existing problems. This seems to supports a stronger call to action to the body. It's like a gentle, persistent nag or reminder that there's work to be done! As a result, some patients feel worse before they begin to feel better. One might be tempted to believe this normal and often-expected homeopathic effect is a Herxheimer reaction. It is absolutely not. Herxheimer reactions are a side effect of antibiotic treatment that results from sudden release of bacterial toxins into the bloodstream. The intense feeling of one's condition worsening is due to inflammation caused by the pharmaceutical intervention. This is known to many as rapid die-off toxicity.

Bio-energetic supplementation wellness support does not kill *anything*, nor does it cause unnatural rapid die-off of bacteria. With the *Bio-energetic Individual Therapy Equation*, one's <u>immune system</u> is the <u>only</u> force for killing bacteria or other microbes. Yes, one may briefly feel worse before feeling better, due to the healing crisis elicited by the homeopathic effect. This can also be the case for symptoms completely unrelated to Lyme disease.

It cannot be stressed loud enough, often enough, and strong enough that there are **NO** side effects from homeopathic energy medicine supplements. They are NOT pharmaceutical drugs, nor are they herbal medications. There is absolutely no <u>chemical</u> effect that can cause any interactions with any medication (over-the-counter or prescribed). They cannot *make* one's body do anything it should not or could not do naturally on its own. If they could, I would not be using them personally or professionally!

"I had muscle and joint pain, bacterial infections, sinus infections and allergies, and Lyme disease. It was difficult to do every day thing such as taking a walk, going to gym and exercise, going dancing, and doing house work. I felt terrible, tired and irritable. I saw many specialists, such as Ear, Nose, and Throat doctors, and Allergy Specialists. I took allergy shots for four years, as well as acupuncture, reflexology and Reiki. Every 3-4 months, I had to take antibiotics of all kinds for all of the last 13 years.... and nothing had been working. In just 4 short months of Dr. Liebell's treatment, I feel alive again. Most all of joint and muscle pain is gone. Allergies and sinus infections are much improved. I am now able to do all of the things I could not do before. Dr. Liebell and his staff listened, and took great amount time to find out about my symptoms, and treated me like family. Dr. Liebell took time to run tests on me that no other specialists had done. The ear acupuncture [Auricular Therapy] feels like a little pinch, no pain at all. He showed me a way to treat all my symptoms without common prescription drugs, and without antibiotics—which has destroyed my entire immune system! He is now treating me with homeopathic supplements. He has improved my health in 4 short months, while no other special has been able to do in 13 years. If it was not for Dr. Liebell, I do believe, my health would have deteriorated further and I would not be able to walk. He is my savior. You have no idea how simple and easy the treatment is, and your health will improve greatly without drugs and antibiotics. There are other choices in life, but no-one tells you about them—because there is no money in it for them. My experience has been wonderful... the best thing I ever did in my life. It saved my life."
- Sandra M., Virginia Beach

Part Five:

Diffusing the Doubters, Detractors, and Disparagers

"The origin of an original work is always the pursuit of a fact which does not fit into accepted ideas"

- Claude Bernard, M.D. (1813-1878): French physician considered as one of the greatest of scientists

Chapter 30

Discernment: Who Are the Kooks And Charlatans?

The American mainstream medical establishment has long portrayed itself as being dedicated to the health of nation's people. Many well-researched books and articles have been written that tear apart the seemingly regal and untouchable institution known as conventional Western medicine. This book is not intended to replace these outstanding publications that have provided convincing evidence that our leading medical organization is dedicated to doctors' wealth more than our health. I wish it were unnecessary for me to even bring any of this up because my mission is to bring a message of realistic hope, encouragement, and enlightenment. However, because mainstream medicine has, for well over one hundred years brutally and savagely done everything in its power to denigrate and demonize any competing health science, philosophy, and art, I must discuss its significance in relation to the *Bio-energetic Individual Treatment Equation©*. Two major components of it, homeopathy and chiropractic, have been long attacked and nearly annihilated by the American Medical Association.

The question I put forth to readers and prospective patients (especially in light of how mainstream medicine addresses tick-triggered illness) is, haven't *they* been given more than a fair chance to prove themselves experts? I also ask, is it unreasonable to question the motives, intent, methods, philosophy, and results of the medical conglomerate that supported the tobacco industry just a few decades ago? The same *trusted* iconic institution that created and approved drugs that have killed more Americans than any war?

We natural and holistic doctors are long tired of having to defend ourselves against the monopolizing and menacing maniacs notorious for convincing the public to enthusiastically take deadly drugs like Vioxx (60,000 known deaths), diet pills like Fen-Phen (estimated over 50,000 lawsuits!), and countless other experimental agents of biochemical mayhem. The public has been duped through decades of brilliantly conceived marketing that mainstream medicine is always scientific and correct. Therefore anything alternative or complementary is unscientific, and must not only be mistrusted, but avoided like the plague for the sake of public safety. So if anybody has any criticism for *my* treatment methods, I can succinctly respond by saying, *"Are you kidding me?"*

I remind you that this book is not a how to guide. Some of the critics of alternative medicine are justified in concerns for people self-treating. The *Bio-energetic Individual Treatment Equation*© is not do-it-yourself treatment. It is a matter of qualified doctor evaluation, treatment, and recommendations. This is a book of hope—not a microbiology, biochemistry, or pathology textbook. I make no medical claims, nor do I deny that I cannot fully prove my patients' results and how they were achieved. In all fairness to me, I see no evidence of anybody else really proving anything either.

"Antibiotics worked for a short time and finally not at all. I had to try something different. Thus, when starting I stuck to [Dr. Liebell's] exact instructions, heeding the fact that there would not be instant success. Today everyone is looking for a fast fix. "I want my hamburger now." "I don't want to wait for fuel in this line. I'll pay more over there." The fast fix is embedded in people's philosophy of life… I have worked in agriculture all my life in a 2 acre greenhouse and also outside in fields producing cut flowers for the retail industry. I have been bitten by every insect I think there is and in the past 30 years contacted Lyme disease. My symptoms included: stiff neck, major joints hurting, feeling languid – basically a loss of energy, a loss of being able to recall names, headaches, and the worst condition - seizures while sleeping leaving me with clouded thinking… I was alerted by others to fact I could probably have Lyme disease because of all the insect contact I have had in my life. I went to a local doctor who specialized in Lyme's only because he contacted it himself in his grape vineyard. He took one look at me and confirmed through tests that I had Lyme's. My symptoms confirmed I have had it for years and that it had settled in my nerve cells. He felt it probably was causing my seizures. He prescribed heavy doses of antibiotics for 3 months. Boy did I feel better. Six months later I was fighting the same symptoms as before. I took more antibiotics and made me feel better again. Evidently the Lyme bacteria were hiding in my head and would precipitate out into the rest of my body in intervals of time. My doctor helped but did not cure the problem. He also retired leaving me without help again. I needed help. My problems were returning again. I found Dr. Liebell's website and decided to try his homeopathic treatment to try to get my body to fight this disease from my own immune system which had become complacent and inoperable… By building my immune system I feel as if my own body is now working to conquer this problem. Many of my problems have been rectified. I am still fighting a stiff neck [severe joint and disc degeneration unrelated to Lyme]. He is a doctor who wishes to cure not just put a band-aid on the problem."

\- Tom Z., Cape Charles, Virginia

Nothing to Hide... Nothing to Defend

It has been well-publicized that medical errors are among the leading causes of death in America. Hundreds of thousands of preventable side effects are experienced every year—mostly from *correctly* prescribed drugs. Millions of people get infections in hospitals—many of them fatal. With tens of thousands of problems occurring daily due to conventional medical care, I feel no compulsion whatsoever to be defensive about my *un*conventional health care services. I have no qualms whatsoever about admitting that nearly every component of the *Bio-energetic Individual Treatment Equation©* is misunderstood and criticized by American mainstream medicine. The biggest criticism seems to be that the methods couldn't possibly work. So much energy wasted, and so much fruitless effort has been made to try to disprove that people can get well without drugs. Is there any other society that performs more excessive risky medical treatment (with appalling statistics) and so shabbily treats those who try other safer, cheaper, and effective methods?

"Been There... Done That... Got the T-Shirt!"

I have never, nor would I ever suggest, insinuate, or order any patient to avoid conventional medical evaluation for Lyme disease. The reality is that 99 percent of patients I see have already had intensive medical evaluation and treatment prior to entering the Liebell Clinic. Since 1993, I've treated numerous people who had failed spinal fusion surgery prior to seeing me for *successful* non-surgical care. These people typically had x-rays, MRIs, CT scans, blood tests, and nerve tests. Prescription painkillers and anti-inflammatory drugs were gulped down without batting an eye. Many had suffered the drudgery of months of physical therapy—ultimately ending up going under the knife, to no avail. This is another example of mainstream medicine poisoning the minds of the public such that they believe expertise can come only in the form of *their* methods.

250

I am by no means suggesting my system is the only effective one. Nobody likes to admit making poor choices. But it seems people tend to cling to them, despite the outcome especially when large amounts of money have been spent. Patients commonly enter the Liebell Clinic hoisting a bag full of vitamins and mineral supplements, herbs, enzymes, antioxidants, and other pills. The patients don't know what to do with them— they've paid for them, but they have not been helping much at all. Often is the case that the patient has been taking their supplements for *years*—and do not feel comfortable without them.

What to Do When People in Your Life Do Not Belief You are Sick

When somebody is suffering many symptoms, but doctors consistently tell family members that nothing wrong can be found—it is the *patient* whose story is doubted. Spouses often hear doctor after doctor say there is no Lyme disease or anything else. Whom do the spouses start to believe…the professionals with all of the medical degrees, credentials, and experience? Or will they believe the suffering patient?

It would not seem terribly unreasonable for a Lyme victim's family to believe the problems are psychiatric in origin. In absence of concrete evidence (by conventional medical standards) the conclusion is psychosomatic, meaning all in the head. Many of my patients have been dismissed as nut cases by doctors, as well as family and friends. The stress of being ostracized only complicates and magnifies the illness. I have found that when patients in this situation recover under my care—they experience an unexpected shock: nobody believes that they are well! In fact, I have seen patients get told that their claim that they have gotten well was proof of being crazy in the first place!

251

When chemical medicine intake results in eliminating symptoms—the *medicine* seems to always get the credit. When a human being naturally heals through the aid of homeopathy or other drugless support, it was the placebo effect or the patient was a nut. What should you do if people do not believe you are sick? My advice is simply to stop caring what these people think! Do not waste your energy trying to convince these people of anything. Save your energy for improving your health. And when you get better...do not bother telling the naysayers. They didn't believe you were really sick in the first place...so why would they believe you have gotten well? Would such people likely believe bio-energetic medicine was the key? I highly doubt it. My advice is to get well, enjoy your life, and only share your experience with those who are open-minded, or truly understand what you've gone through. Save your energy for those who need help too, and can benefit from your success story.

Why is the *Bio-Energetic Individual Treatment Equation* Not Being Studied by Mainstream Medicine?

Authentic natural healing cannot be traded on the New York Stock Exchange. It is not a commodity for sale as pharmaceutical medicines are. Auricular therapy and upper cervical chiropractic are low-cost health services. Homeopathic bio-energetic supplements are inexpensive and non-addictive. They cannot be patented either. The formulas themselves are intellectual property—like a copyright. Dr. Nader Soliman has created many amazing health supports. They are produced by the company, Homeodynamics based out of Wisconsin. These products have never been, nor will they ever be marketed as cures or direct medical treatments for any illness. They will not be studied by mainstream medicine because they do not fit the conventional medical model.

In May of 2014 I attended a unique event that was held at *Johns Hopkins University* in Maryland. It was the *Eighth International Symposium of Auriculotherapy*. This was a 3-day educational gathering of doctors and acupuncturists who utilize auricular therapy (ear acupuncture) methods. Those who have performed it know the fantastic results it can achieve. For us, it is not *alternative* to anything. It is not a last resort, but rather often the first defense! You would be very surprised at some of the academic medical credentials of the symposium attendees.

The BITE is NOT Represented as a Replacement for Your Conventional Family Physician

The task at hand is to provide wellness support, as well as drugless and non-surgical pain relief options. I am extremely proud of what I do. However, no doctors trained in this system position their services as a replacement for conventional medical diagnosis and treatment. The BITE can be utilized in conjunction with, or instead of them, by the choice of the patient.

Integrative Medicine: 21st Century Health Care

I am a supporter of integrative medicine. This means that ALL methods, philosophies, and treatment approaches are considered for the benefit of patients. I personally practice holistic methods that are drugless and non-surgical. This does not imply that I think drugs and surgery are unnecessary or fundamentally bad. On the contrary, I am in awe of many conventional medical practices. What I am staunchly opposed to is closed-mindedness, laziness, ignorance, and greed. I am in favor of putting patients' needs before profits.

I think the term integrative is unnecessary. Medicine is medicine! The word itself comes from Latin, *ars medicina*, which means the art of healing. All health care practices are for the purposes of improving health. In practice, I do not separate health care into different factions. There is a time and a place for the different types of treatment and diagnostic approaches.

I prefer treatment methods that are natural, and have a scientific basis. This is not to say that all treatments that don't stand up to peer-reviewed academic medical research standards or conditions are invalid. Not everything can be tested sufficiently in a double-blind research study. The human body is capable of healing in ways science does not fully understand. There are methods that are highly effective, but are so customized to the individual (rather than a disease) that it doesn't fit the model of standard research.

The fact remains that there are many highly effective, scientifically proven alternatives to drugs and surgery that are used throughout the world. These days, more Americans are seeking mainstream medicine for diagnostic testing with the intention of pursuing natural and holistic treatments. This is known as an integrated medical approach because it is a combination of conventional medical treatments with complementary or alternative approaches. In my opinion, it is critical to neither reject all conventional Western medicine, nor uncritically accept all alternative medicine. Medical treatment should be designed to fit the needs of the individual patient, with consideration for any and all approaches.

Health care methods beyond the realm of the American pharmaceutical model are typically lumped into the category of alternative medicine. This is shameful. Despite the obscene amount of money Americans spend on health care, we are far from the healthiest people in the world. My mission is to be a leader in an American upgrade! With an integrated medical approach, we consider the BIG Picture. The patient's individual and complete story is of the utmost importance—not just a symptom or diagnosis. Our bodies are composed of many integrated systems. Pain and other symptoms often have more than just one cause. Therefore, problems often require more than just one treatment approach. The key is to treat PEOPLE, not medical conditions. There is a colossal difference. Each person must be evaluated and treated as a unique whole—an integrated system that can have multiple blockages or interferences to normal function (homeostasis).

The ordinary doctor regards the patient's symptoms and perhaps some test findings, and writes a prescription or two. The *extraordinary* doctor ferrets out the reasons the person's body is not functioning, and develops the best strategy to restore function—to naturally eliminate symptoms and promote better health. No stone can be left unturned when it comes to your health. The key is to get behind the causes of your symptoms and provide your body with the missing tools it needs to defend against it. Lifestyle factors, injuries, and diet each have an impact on your individual situation. You can't go back in time and change the past, but you can promote a better, healthier future right now. While it is nice that international science supports many so-called complementary and alternative medicine procedures, the bottom line is that great *results* and patient satisfaction supports them.

Instead of merely naming or labeling your condition (diagnosis), the bulk of our effort goes into answering critical questions such as:

> ➤ What and where are the CAUSES of the symptom?
> ➤ Is that location a PRIMARY focus? Or is it secondary to another cause somewhere else in the body?
> ➤ What is making this problem chronic?
> ➤ Is it a structural problem?
> ➤ Is it a neurological problem?
> ➤ Are there energetic disturbances or blockages?
> ➤ Are there nutritional problems?

- What other areas and systems of the body are involved?
- What can be done to break the cycle of dysfunction that the patient is stuck in?
- What types of treatment are likely to be most helpful?
- Does your case require the expertise of other physicians or diagnostic tests?

Obviously a whole new diagnosis and treatment perspective is required to answer these questions. We need the whole story, not just the basic surface facts—the symptoms. Investigation of the various imbalances within the body is the key to discovering, and properly treating the underlying causes of pain and disease. The integrative approach is clearly the most advanced, scientific and complete model of health care possible. Plus, it is not the property of any faction of health care. It is neither alternative nor conventional. It is a comprehensive model of health care that requires doctors to think critically. With a cooperative spirit, it requires doctors of every discipline to be open-minded and informed, and to be receptive to various treatment methods—not just their own specialty. When doctors of all disciplines learn to recognize this, the most effective treatment plans can be created. These are treatment plans that consider multiple approaches and options. These are treatment plans that integrate the healing arts, philosophies and science from around the world.

In the integrated medical world, practitioners are equal and important, whether they are a traditional medical doctor, chiropractor, neurosurgeon, naturopath, osteopath, herbalist, acupuncturist, etc. We recognize the need for every type of practitioner and method to help people get better and stay better—all without the interferences of personal ego…without attitudes of superiority, and most importantly without ignorance of the methods of others. We doctors must evaluate patients and select the appropriate treatment methods from a greatly expanded toolkit.

256

Pain Motivation Mishaps

It's tough to think clearly when you're in pain. That's why millions of Americans seek the fastest pain relief they can get their hands on—and maybe think about side effects later, if at all. The pharmaceutical companies understand this psychology all too well. It's easy to believe what the drug commercials say. They are quite skillful at painting a wonderful picture—a world that's free of pain, suffering and disease. Their commercials are packed with beautiful pictures, emotional music, attractive people, and a grand message of hope. The problem is that they are selling an illusion of health, not the reality.

Obviously, there are times that drugs can save your life, or get you through a painful crisis. The fundamental principle of conventional Western medicinal pain treatment is to block or suppress pain signals with drugs. I appreciate and applaud medical developments to make this possible. However, isn't it a loftier goal to enable true healing—to promote your body's ability to eliminate pain without drugs? I <u>never</u> advise patients to cease taking medication (they do that on their own when appropriate, in conjunction with the prescribing physician). In my practice, I seek only methods that un-block interference to the body's energetic systems.

The True Middle Ground in Medicine

The public has been well-exposed to sources intent on scaring the public away from so-called alternative medicine. Their premise is that there can be only one king, who rules over health care—the *American Medical Association*. By their standards, any other way of doing things is wrong. This closed-minded thinking works both ways. Alternative medicine practitioners who bash everything in conventional medicine are equally prejudiced. Even though the death toll from Western medicine warrants some bias, it would be foolhardy to avoid it as a whole.

The advances in health care that have drastically improved the quality of human life cannot be underestimated. This does not however, give Western medicine a free pass to do whatever it wants without scrutiny. No medical system is perfect. This is the case for both conventional Western medical testing and treatment, as well as all other methods.

One of the flaws of Western medicine with chronic illness is its focus on the condition rather than the individual. There is no standard drug for an individual. One size does not fit all. The conventional medical establishment has been stunningly convincing that every illness or symptom is something that requires treatment with a specific drug. They have also made consistent and calculated efforts to suppress any health care methods outside of that realm. The *natural* health community, on the other hand, suggests that illness is mostly the result of poor lifestyle choices. This usually refers to diet and exercise. I say both medical viewpoints are dead wrong! They are equally too extreme to be accurate. Health is not black and white. The practice of prescribing a drug for every symptom as a means of health care is tragic on so many levels. The fact is the natural health advocates are oversimplifying things too. It is equally untrue that *everything* that goes wrong in your body is the result of lifestyle choices. Diet and exercise is not the answer to everything either, nor are processed nutritional supplements and herbs. Websites, books, and other publications that regularly promote a conspiracy theory type of outlook on mainstream medicine, are in my opinion, taking the same low road. They too often radically oppose mainstream medicine as vehemently as seen with American partisan politics.

Is it important for you to make healthy choices? Of course it is. Statistically speaking, Americans are not a healthy bunch. More than half the deaths in the U.S. result from chronic illness— many of which are preventable. Sure, most Americans eat a poor diet and are overweight. Avoiding genetically modified

258

foods (GMOs) is a great idea. You should indeed eat as much organic produce as possible, including more raw vegetables. Keeping your home free of unnecessary chemicals from cleaners, air fresheners, fabric softeners, and dozens of home products would be brilliant. Yes, toxic chemicals, smoking, excessive alcohol consumption, processed junk foods, and other factors are major contributors in the deterioration of health.

But…

None of these things cause people to be bitten by ticks, mosquitoes, flies, mites, and other wretched "buggy" life forms—and to be infected by what they transmit!

The *Bio-energetic Individual Treatment Equation©* functions on the middle ground between the two opposite factions in health care. While I stand firm with our holistic treatment philosophy, we acknowledge infectious microbes (germs) as agents of pain and illness—perhaps even *more* so than the medical mainstream currently does publicly. Medical journals are overflowing with published papers that relate common health problems to viruses, bacteria, and other microbes. The public knows that germs are agents of disease. However, the actual clinical practice of medicine lacks focus on this microscopic world beyond rampant antibiotic prescription. The microbial causes of disease are highly-acknowledged in *academic medical publication*—but scarcely in clinical diagnosis and treatment. Using the bio-energetic techniques described in this book to investigate the association between germs and illness, we can bridge the gap.

"Esma suffered deep aches in her muscles and bones, confusion, fatigue, weakness, nausea, blurred vision, and weird sensations in her head. She went to many specialists. At times I had to carry her into the emergency room. I was desperate and panicked. The doctors never told us anything. Lyme tests were negative, but eventually a doctor told us Esma had a tumor of the pituitary gland in her brain. Only 42 years old, with a beautiful heart, I wanted to help her so much. I couldn't sleep constantly thinking of what I could do to help heal her. I read Dr. Liebell's website and liked his commitment to healing people and his approach. When Esma had her very first visit with Dr. Liebell, we did not know what to expect, other than praying that he will be the one doctor who will help her. Walking into the office, the office staff are so kind and caring which was very comforting to Esma and me, compared to what we have been through. For the first time in months we finally had confirmation of what was wrong with her health...that alone was a huge accomplishment.

Esma started her homeopathic protocol. Dr. Liebell told us that Esma might feel worse, and then she will start feeling better. He was spot on with this...feeling worse was a good sign—it meant the homeopathy medicine was working, and her body was detoxifying. Esma is now cured 100% from the chronic Lyme disease. Her proof of that is no more anxiety....no more deep pain in her joints... no more ache in her muscles...no more low grade fever...no more getting out of bed in the morning—taking her almost 2 hours to be able to walk ok....no more shortness of breath when walking up steps...no more unknown bumps in her back...all of those symptoms are gone. Esma and I cannot put in words our gratitude and appreciation of his dedication and compassion that he has showed her from day one and still does...her experience with the doctor and his staff is an experience she will think of each day when she gets out of bed and can walk with no pain... can run the steps now with no shortness of breath... And can actually go to sleep at night time. We cannot express how much we care about and respect Dr. Liebell. He is the kind of doctor who we have not ever experienced such dedication, caring, and compassion for his patients...a blessing he is."
     - Jeff G. and Esma T., Virginia Beach

"Anthropology demands the open-mindedness with which one must look and listen, record in astonishment and wonder that which one would not have been able to guess." — Margaret Mead

Chapter 31

Putting Placebo Proclaimers in Their Place

Why Cries of "Placebo Effect" Do Not Hold Water

It would come as no great surprise for the *Bio-energetic Individual Treatment Equation*© to receive criticism. My suspicion is that the loudest cries would come from those who have never helped a single victim of tick-triggered illness get well in their lives. Some might come from antibiotic-focused doctors, who have no experience with authentic natural healing, and thus do not believe people can get well without drugs. I would also not be shocked to hear accusations of quackery or the placebo effect. I do not wish to waste time with an ongoing discussion to *defend* the means by which *Bio-Energetic Individual Treatment Equation* patients achieve magnificent results. I have written this chapter to get this topic out of the way, and put it to bed once and for all. There are some individuals (I will not mention names and play *their* slanderous games) who have made it their mission to discredit any and all health care measures that do not fall within the confines of the accepted practices of American conventional medicine. They often blabber that when natural methods work—it is because the ailment was self-limiting, meaning that it would have gone away itself anyway. More insulting to us out-of-the-box thinking, hard-working, caring, and holistic-minded doctors is the suggestion that any results our patients obtain are due to the placebo effect. In other words, our procedures do not actually do anything for the patient—it is just mind over matter.

Holistic doctors are sometimes accused of gaining large followings of patients because of their extraordinary *kindness* and *compassion*. The implication is that we do not actually provide any tangible treatment. These loathsome critics grumble that we have no business taking credit for the results of our treatment. Odd it is that when it comes to prescription medication and surgery, all bets are off! The *real* medicine is always responsible for the results. How pompous it is to warn consumers to be leery of natural and holistic health care methods when so-called scientific pharmaceutical medicine is among the leading causes of death in America! The despicable self-appointed crusaders against quackery insist that when people testify to results of any *alternative* medicine—it was the body's own natural healing power that was responsible for the cure rather than the treatment. The double standard these crumbs maintain is astonishing. How badly they miss the boat. The whole point of most natural methods *is* to enable the body to heal itself. We have always given the credit to the innate healing capacity of the human body!

"I was diagnosed with Lyme disease in 1991, and have had several flare-ups since. I read about Dr. Liebell and his work with Lyme disease and homeopathic treatments. Making an appointment with him was one of the best decisions I've made. At my first appointment, I was using a cane to walk and had much pain in my legs, along with many other symptoms that come with Lyme. Dr. Liebell treated me as an individual and treated each of my symptoms. Homeopathy definitely works. I feel better now than I have in many years." - Teresa B., Virginia Beach, VA

Bitter, jealous, and ignorant critics of natural health methods are obsessed with rival methods that equal or outperform pharmaceutical medicine and surgery. I have little doubt that unscrupulous shills for greedy drug companies are paid to write articles to try to discredit any competition. One obnoxious doctor's article suggested that post-treatment Lyme disease syndrome patients only improve under holistic care merely because they *believe* the treatment will help. This critic also boasts that patients get better because somebody is *finally* taking their symptoms seriously. I wonder if these misguided fools even realize how stupid they sound when they intentionally point out that conventional medical doctors (the supposedly *scientific* practitioners) may not take their patients seriously. Wow!

By the time patients wind up in my office, they typically have been through many other treatment protocols for which they too had high hopes for success. They were assured by the high authorities, including rheumatologists, neurologists, infectious disease specialists, and family practitioners that medications such as doxycycline and others drugs would cure them. Their expectations must certainly have been high, since they were presented with supposedly the ultimate care from established credible scientific medicine. **Where was the placebo effect then?**

Many long-suffering patients have reported that despite being assured of a cure, they failed to improve with the medically-accepted duration of antibiotic treatment. Next, they pursued aggressive long-term antibiotic protocols from doctors who acknowledge chronic Lyme disease. The results were no better. The doctors certainly presented the patients with a pedigree of expertise, credentials, and confidence in their methods. **Why wasn't the placebo effect anywhere to be found?**

Still other patients failed to get better after standard conventional medical and extreme conventional methods were exhausted. They turned to Rife machines, herbal protocols, diets, cleanses, nutritional supplements, and other so-called alternative medicine approaches. They stood in the presence of those presumably more caring practitioners. Surely with money being spent on treatment *not* covered by insurance, they were even more motivated to succeed. The mind-over-matter factor was in full force, wasn't it?

"Elvis has left the building"...
along with the legendary placebo effect!

The insufferable enemies of natural healing disapprove of our methods. They pass judgment with the unsubstantiated claim that we are unscientific healers that do not conform to the values of reputable medicine. Arrogant cynics assert that real doctors do not rely on the *simplicity* of nature as their cure. They view their methods as complex and therefore superior. Simplicity of nature? Patients who frequent the Liebell Clinic are rarely folks afflicted with minor problems that would naturally work their way out if given time. With the debilitating chronic ailments associated with tick-borne infection (as well as upper cervical spine dysfunction), we are not talking about a common cold going away itself whether medicated or not. The power of suggestion is not the mechanism of cure. The cure comes from within—relying on the awe-inspiring *complexity* of nature. Patient recovery is due to the incredible healing power of the human body—given extraordinarily effective support!

"Isn't the Effect Just Mind-Over-Matter?"

This is a dull and tiresome argument that closed-minded pharmaceutical-minded doctors love to cry in criticism of their extraordinarily safe and inexpensive competitors. There is much evidence that their accusations are unfounded and, in my opinion slanderous. For example, in 1997, the well-respected medical journal, the *Lancet* published a comprehensive analysis of 89 separate studies on homeopathy for various illnesses. They concluded that homeopathy's effectiveness was NOT from the placebo effect. What about all the babies and small children worldwide, who have been helped by homeopathy? Was there a placebo effect for them? Of course the most stunning defeat of the idea comes from the fact that homeopathy has been successfully used for animals!

Critics of homeopathic medicine say it is not an acceptable therapy because it has not been validated by large-scale, double-blind, placebo controlled medical studies. This argument does not hold water because this is also true for most mainstream medical procedures and drugs! Various sources say maybe 10-20 percent of accepted conventional medical practices can legitimately claim they've been really proven. As mentioned frequently throughout this book, it is not even known how a solid percentage of the FDA-approved prescription medications actually work!! What sad commentary it is to call people who testify to their success with holistic natural treatments as quackery victims who were hoodwinked by the placebo effect or coincidence. How pathetic it is to hassle and hound doctors who successfully guide their long-suffering patients back to health—without a single drop of chemical medicine. The people seeking help are not the ones who cry placebo, but rather the fearful conventional medical establishment. Their financial and political agendas are threatened by safe, inexpensive, and effective health care.

The crusaders for chemical conventional medicine are the ones likely asking, "Dr. Liebell, don't your patients really just get better because of the power of suggestion?" "Come on, doctor… you are so positive, caring, kind, and motivating— don't you think *that* is why your patients succeed after others have failed?" "Seriously doctor, you take so much time to explain things—to educate patients about how the human body works, and what enhances health… isn't *that* why your patients get well? It couldn't really be your treatment, could it?" "Dr. Liebell, aren't your patients so desperate for help that they'll try *anything*? Isn't their wishful thinking at its peak?"

I wish it *were* that easy! If all I ever had to do to help people with supposedly hopeless cases of chronic pain and illness was to be caring and loving, I would have saved a fortune earning bachelor's, doctoral and post-doctoral degrees, and equipping an office with treatment technologies. Technically a placebo effect is a positive response to any procedure, device, treatment, or substance that cannot be explained by pharmacology or physical action. The patient *expects* it to work, so sometimes it does. Overall, I must say that the most infuriating attack comes in the form of lambasting successful natural health practitioners for having charismatic personalities. Should a doctor feel apologetic for having a pleasing personality, a great bedside manner, or for exuding confidence and caring?

Seriously? The reality is that my typical patient is <u>not</u> enthusiastic or high in expectations. It is quite the contrary. Most new patients are in fact, highly skeptical, very troubled, and distrustful of doctors due to previous experience. They have spent fortunes on care that failed. What a thrill it is to see them blossom back to health. These folks are 100% certain their recovery was not due to their expectations, since they had none!

"I too had Lyme disease. After many attempts from conventional medicine, nothing worked. I was told it was in my head and that I was completely healthy. Only the people who've had Lyme know the pain and complications this debilitating disease can cause. It will destroy you in every aspect. After six months of antibiotics one after the other I was told there was nothing they could do that maybe I should try alternative medicine. That's where Dr. Liebell comes in. I found his website after searching for

what seemed like months. At first I was skeptical but didn't know what else to do or turn. So I took the three hour drive to his office and got his protocol but I was still skeptical. After about 2 months I knew it was working, so I continued with his protocol. The thing about Lyme there is no funding for research of this disease and the cost of antibiotics are real expensive even with insurance and after a while, they don't want to pay anymore because the CDC doesn't acknowledge chronic Lyme disease. Dr. Liebell has helped me tremendously along with other family and friends. One family member went to him skeptical just like me but did the protocol and returned to their conventional doctor to be told their health was getting better not knowing they were doing Dr. Liebell's protocol and not the prescriptions. That was the proof in the pudding. I thank GOD every time I pray for leading me to him. Thanks Dr. Liebell."

- Keith S., Gordonsville, VA

The placebo effect is a real phenomenon. Some people are more likely to be influenced by expectations than others. Perhaps those folks are more likely to respond favorably to *any* treatment. However, that is not the type of person who seeks my care. I see the people for whom any potential placebo effect has been long extinguished. Everything else had already failed regardless of the doctors' confidence or the patients' expectations. I would again ask any critic, where was the placebo effect during all of the previous treatments provided by both conventional and alternative practitioners?

Frankly, I don't care whether or not any patient gets well via the placebo effect… as long as they get well. Belief and expectations for treatment success can only help, but they are not required if the method is truly good. The *Bio-energetic Individual Treatment Equation©* works beautifully regardless of your belief in its likely effectiveness. I can assure you that I've been faced with way more people who were skeptical and negative, than those who had high expectations… and prevailed regardless.

267

Pride and Prejudice

While writing this book, I have been aware that many doctors may be prejudiced against me, our cause, and methods, before even giving the topic reasonable thought. There are those who have it set in their minds that disease can only be fought through pharmaceutical intervention endorsed and created in conjunction with the *American Medical Association* (AMA). Perhaps these professionals need reminding that we are all human beings with the capacity to care for one another. There have been numerous methods of health care used throughout history and around the world that have merit. While the *business* of medicine has unfortunately deteriorated into a ruthless dog-eat-dog competition for the consumer dollar—health *care* has been, and will always be about guiding patients towards better health. I humbly implore those who are prejudiced against alternative medicine to put their biases aside (at least temporarily) and carefully consider the contents of this book. One of my goals is to teach other doctors—so the masses can be helped.

I make no brash, bold, or controversial statement by proclaiming that chronic pain and illness can consistently be resolved without a single molecule of pharmaceutical chemical medicine. Highly-educated medical professionals, with all of their profound and complex learning—all of their cumulative knowledge of biochemistry, molecular biology, etc. should realize that I am not claiming any miraculous skill or ability unique to myself. The skills and knowledge I possess have been available to those who are willing to pursue such training. Thought, desire, and perseverance have been the only requirements.

Drugs and surgery are *perceived* by both the general public and conventionally-trained American medical doctors as the normal, legitimate, scientific, and appropriate means of treating human ills. *Perception* is the operative word. Throughout every period in human history there has always been a perception of what is *correct*, appropriate or normal. What has put the "conventional" in conventional Western medicine has been a calculated, well-funded, and ruthless effort to craft and mold public opinion. For several generations in America, the perception has been that chemical medicine is the real medicine. Any method or system that differs from the pharmaceutical mindset is medical heresy, insultingly labeled alternative medicine. The public has embraced this inaccurate terminology, perhaps not contemplating that many of the methods that fall under its umbrella existed ages before the current conventional practices. These alternative methods may outlive them too.

If it Quacks Like a Duck...

Drug-based medicine has been fashionable for some time. It has held a mental monopoly in the minds of Americans such that anybody who practices differently, or questions its authority is an unscientific quack. Although interpretation of the definition of the term, quackery varies, it implies unproven or fraudulent medical practices. A quack pretends to possess skill or knowledge—a phony. Today the term, pseudoscience, is more popular to tarnish the reputation of any unconventional healing art. Frightened bullies, who have never mastered *any* of the methods they lambast, insist they are not actually effective, but merely claim to be. It is fascinating how these critics appoint themselves authorities on subjects for which they have no actual experience or knowledge, but are certain of their opinion. What constitutes science may be as polarized as politics. How does one determine the acceptable standard for effectiveness of medicine? The *American Medical Association*? This biased doctors' lobbyist organization has a rich history of doing everything in their power to eliminate any competition to their financial monopoly on American health care.

There is a level of uncertainty with all medical treatments. What matters is what claims are being made, as well as safety. There are those who misrepresent the nature of the treatments, or the risks and benefits. The highest of established medical authorities surely admit medicine is an imperfect science. There is no denying the risks of deadly side effects. It isn't called the *practice* of medicine for nothing! It is an ongoing and necessary experiment. Those potentially deadly risks must be disclosed with pharmaceutical advertising. Of course, those side effects are fine print or fast talk, typically advertised as rare.
Many an honorable physician has fled their profession in detestable disgust to many of its practices. I believe more would eagerly follow in their footsteps—if they could be assured of making the same or better living by alternative means. I am far from alone in the field of health care, who consider the overuse and abuse of drug treatments as one of the keys to the deterioration and decline of health. But as long as those who are in power justify the accepted standard of health care to be patients swallowing drugs for every imaginable symptom— natural healing arts will be overlooked, ridiculed, mocked, and belittled by the masses. The fault lies however, in not only the doctors, drug companies, their lobbyists and sales representatives, but the public's unquestioning trust in their safety and effectiveness. Consumers must not be blindly subservient to the authority of mainstream medicine.

True health is when the human body's systems, organs, glands, tissues, cells, etc. are performing their normal functions. That is what we call normal physiology. The self-important, self-appointed health authorities seem to suggest that there is no common ground. The human body is treated by AMA standards of care, and that's that. There is no compromise. Any other means to ensure better health is unscrupulously labeled quackery—even though it is firmly acknowledged that medicine can never truly be a pure science.

The term quackery, by the way, refers to someone who professes health care knowledge for which he or she lacks scientific qualifications. The word quack is short for *quacksalver*—derived from a Dutch word which means to boast. To boast means to speak with excessive pride and self-satisfaction about one's achievements, possessions, or abilities. And excessive means beyond what is necessary, normal, or desired. The conventional medical establishment has certainly *boasted* that doxycycline cures Lyme disease. Have they not been excessive in *their* claims? Ironic it is that Louis Pasteur was initially accused of quackery for suggesting sterilization of food with heat! One of the most vocal critics of alternative medicine—apparently an advisor to various U.S. Government agencies (who shall remain nameless) is an unlicensed physician, who serves as a vigilante to allegedly protect the public!

Human experience cannot be reduced to mathematical equations. No person's health picture is black or white. Doctors cannot tell whether the drug that was prescribed enabled the patient to get well, or if to credit the natural healing power of the patient's body. On the other hand, I *always* credit the body! Anything I do for a patient is geared toward supporting (rather than antagonizing) it. I *never* have claimed credit for any cure or healing. My enthusiasm for the methods I use should never be mistaken for boastful bragging or excessive claims. Passionately heralding the natural healing power of the human body is neither a scientific claim nor a practice of medicine. Speaking out against conventional medical wisdom regarding Lyme disease is neither harmful nor irrational. I do not reject antibiotic or other drug usage for victims of tick-triggered illness because I dislike them, or because it is not within my scope of practice to prescribe them. I have the repeated experience of patients reporting their failure to recover from tick-triggered illness with them. More importantly, I have had the privilege of witnessing consistent restoration of health *without* them! This is not a medical claim. There is nothing boastful or excessive about this fact. Those practitioners who have never experienced the joy of practicing methods which result in the human body naturally healing itself would be unlikely to understand. It is a fact that all kinds of diseases may be curable, however not necessarily to the same degree of recovery for each patient, and certainly not all patients.

The question is, if natural treatments can result in recovery—why has the mainstream of medicine not jumped on the bandwagon? Why are Lyme savvy doctors harping on practices of aggressive chemical intervention—if magnificent results can be achieved naturally? This is a question I cannot answer on their behalf. I can however, reiterate the certainty that medicine is a ruthless and competitive business. It is human nature to try to forge one's own niche. I am known to many as the guru of natural treatment for chronic Lyme disease. I did not appoint myself such a title. Indeed, I whole-heartedly advocate the methods I use, and accordingly have no delusions that those who take different approaches would not promote their own as well.

I am in awe of many of the skills, technologies, and achievements of conventional Western medicine. In fact, I cannot argue that antibiotics are one of the most significant achievements in the history of medicine. How their overuse and abuse has ruined things, is another story. I have written this book to exercise my Constitutional right to freedom of speech. Patients have consistently fled from conventional medical treatment (due to its failure) to seek my natural healing methods. The sad part is that it is usually a last resort—after the tens of thousands of dollars in tests and treatments covered by health insurance have failed to deliver the goods.

A New Perspective for an Old Problem

Taking a patient's temperature and pulse, looking at images of the brain on an MRI, looking at blood test results, etc. does not enable the physician to determine a regimen of bio-energetic treatment. Nor does it give the slightest insight to correcting structural skeletal imbalances. We bite back by taking a different path. Consider different types of engineers—mechanical, electrical, nuclear, etc. Each specialist analyzes things from a different scientific perspective, using their associated skill sets and tools. We bite back at chronic tick-triggered illness by applying *different* sciences to enable patients to restore health. And we are doing so in most cases, after the conventional and many unconventional methods have failed.

There is an endless sea of wonderful books, articles, and speeches that champion the healing power of the human body. This is a wonderful thing. But all of the philosophical talk about the mind-body connection, and all the motivational speeches in the world will not take a stagnant and struggling immune system that is losing the battle against numerous infectious microorganisms and save the day. The purpose of the *Bio-energetic Individual Treatment Equation*© is to take specific action—to finally help human beings who have suffered illness, as well as the humiliation, expense, danger, and futility of being put through the mill of modern medicine. The BITE serves to enable sick and suffering people to unleash the hindered potential of their inborn healing power.

The tragic conventional treatment casualties of apparent tick-triggered illness I have encountered have propelled me into action. My patients motivated me to write this book. Throughout my 23-year adventure witnessing the awe-inspiring and mighty healing ability of the human body, I have learned the importance of sticking with my own gifts, talents, and convictions. Remaining loyal to my patients without ever letting

273

others tempt or persuade me to abandon my principles has enabled wonderful things to happen for those I serve. If the perception is that the results are achieved due to the patient's expectations—the placebo effect, then so be it. Patients do not care one bit. They only care that they got their health restored! And they didn't have to risk side effects or death! Unlike many antibiotic-based doctors and drug companies, I have never been the subject of a lawsuit or state board inquisition for treatment. I don't care what doctors, scientists, politicians, or anybody else think—I'm only interested in helping sick people get well.

Chapter 32

Why Some People Respond Better Than Others

The *Bio-energetic Individual Treatment Equation©* is a means of supporting your body to self-heal. It is NOT self-diagnosis, nor is it self-treatment. All improvement however, is naturally occurring as the direct result of improved physiology. Treatment measures are intended to "open the doors" for your body to overcome chronic infection, toxicity, and damage by means of its own natural inborn capabilities.

I would be dubious of any treatment that professes to work 100% of the time. Some patients simply do not follow treatment instructions. Others insist on doing all kinds of *other* treatments at the same time that put stress on the body. Not every person is willing or able to make the commitment to very gradually getting better. There are patients who start care, but don't follow up for reasons unknown for certain to us. Occasionally, a patient will simply quit because they didn't achieve a quick fix. There will be cases where we felt certain success would be achieved, yet for reasons unknown, it didn't work. There are of course, circumstances where the patient has had significant physical damage that may be beyond natural repair.

I ask my patients (regardless of severity, complexity, and duration of their health problems) to consider the task presented to me: to resolve cases of one of the most difficult problems to help... and to do so after many have failed to get positive results at the hands of some of the biggest names in medicine.... and to do so with absolutely no drugs, or complex and difficult therapy regimens.

275

Everybody has a different capacity for healing from the same types of problems. One never knows how much, how fast, and how soon anybody will respond. The variables of treatment are as unique as each individual. We are not treating a disease; we are treating a PERSON. Some people do take longer than a year, but wouldn't continue to see me if they were not making significant progress. I do not treat Lyme disease in the direct medical sense. I provide natural supportive whole-body, wellness care—to support natural function of the body. I understand that people want to know a success rate. What I can humbly state is approximately 80% of patients report successful self-healing. Let me be clear that I am not making a medical claim or success rate. Patients may state that cure has been achieved. It is their right to do so.

Injuries and Damage

Injuries cause damage. For example, a severe joint sprain or dislocation causes physical and chemical changes to the ligaments involved. The damaged tissues can indeed heal, however they do not repair with the same substance as the original. This is the nature of scar tissue. If you badly injured your knee as a teenager, your susceptibility to future knee problems would increase. As the expression goes, a chain is only as strong as its weakest link. What does this have to do with Lyme disease? Quite a lot. Many recovered Lyme victims often find themselves far less tolerant to many things than they once were. Does this mean they didn't really get well? It does not. What it means is that injury from trauma, chronic infection caused tissue damage. Whatever body systems, specific organs, tissues, or regions were deteriorated or altered by the effects of infection are no different from an old sports injury.

A few years ago, I severely injured my right hand in a fall. The back side of my hand got torn nearly to the bone. Through a variety of treatments, I was able to significantly recover—but not one hundred percent. My skin and tendons over my pinky, as well as my ring, and middle finger were torn up. I have scar tissue which slightly limits my grip strength, and feels stiff. This injury makes my right hand more susceptible to injury than my left hand. It is much more sensitive. This means that new infections or irritants can provoke old symptoms. Yes, it is not fair. In fact, my now vast involvement in the study of the microscopic world has brought new meaning to the axiom, "life is not fair."

The *Borrelia* bacterium is not new—it has been around the world for thousands of years, at the least. Countless microbes have always been transmitted to humans by ticks, mosquitoes, flies, mites, lice, and other bugs. We eat food laden with parasites, large and small. Air is breathed into our lungs, carrying molds, viruses, and millions of chemical particles. It has always been this way. The human immune system has a proven track record of success in handling these irritants, although not everybody has equal abilities. This too is not fair—but it is indeed true.

I have always found math to be difficult, dare I say painful. My school transcripts might give the impression otherwise. The fact is that I had to work extremely hard to get great math grades, and be in honors classes all the way through high school. It seemed like my closest friends were math whiz kids; they made it look so easy. They had extremely high aptitudes for learning and developing math skills. I had to work long and hard to keep up. Math was something I dreaded. I've always thought, boy it would have been great if I could write essays for math—instead of solving problems! Yes, it wasn't fair. But that's life. Some people find math easy, while others never really "get it."

A person can have a burning desire to paint, or play a musical instrument, but not have enough aptitude or physical skill to become a master, no matter how hard he or she tries. The same is true regarding health. Some people can be bitten by ticks and other critters that carry a multitude of microorganisms—but they remain unaffected by them. Their immune systems can deal with certain bacteria, viruses, fungi, or other germs just fine. Others come down with every possible symptom from the slightest exposure. There's no disputing this is not fair either. There are people who don't catch colds or flu, or don't ever get sick in general—yet they get hammered by the microbes injected by a measly tick! Life's not fair.

Think about doctors across the world who are exposed daily to numerous infectious microorganisms from sick people. Do they all catch their patients' illnesses? Mostly, they do not. Why not? It's simple: their immune systems prevent it. If you understand this connection between life's-not-fair susceptibility to illness and the capability of the human immune system to overcome Lyme disease, you are handing yourself the potential key to the castle. It is no stretch of imagination, nor is it remotely unscientific to acknowledge that our immune system alone can defeat Lyme disease and other chronic infection. Just because documentary films spread the message of doom… and just because Lyme-savvy doctors say you need to be bombarded with antibiotics to get the job done, does not make it suddenly untrue.

Over the course of the year, applying the BITE, the patient typically experiences slow, but steady and progressive improvement. Ups and downs are a normal part of life— applying the BITE is no exception. Nevertheless, overcoming chronic pain and illness is taking place by the body's natural mechanisms. The gradual restoration of energy, the reduction in headaches, joint and muscle pains, cognitive difficulties, and

278

other common Lyme-related symptoms is purely the result of self-healing. It is not the illusion of health that is commonly provided by symptom-suppressing drugs and/or herbal and pharmaceutical medication.

It is critical to shed the limiting belief that treatment is only effective if it quickly makes you feel better. Pain pills are popular for good reason. However, the consequences of covering up pain—leaving the actual problems unchanged are dire. It is essential to come to grips with the *Bio-Energetic Individual Treatment Equation©* as a health and wellness process—not a pain management or bacteria-killing treatment.

When a professional athlete suffers an injury such as a ligament tear, rehabilitation is typically a difficult, lengthy, and often painful process. The athlete does not expect to be cured of an injury without significant challenge. This includes both breakthroughs and setbacks. Consider the monumental undertaking it is for a chronically ill body to recover—really improve, without drugs… without having to cycle on and off different antibiotics. To overcome viruses, fungi, and parasites for which no treating drugs exist. Just imagine the complex rehab your body must accomplish on a cellular level.

"After years of seeking medical help and getting nowhere, I saw Dr. Liebell and am finally on the road to recovery. Dr. Liebell is a genius and I can't recommend his treatment highly enough. His staff responds to your concerns in a professional, caring and compassionate manner, and they are committed to your recovery from this terrible disease. Dr. Liebell is a treasure. We are so fortunate to have him in our community. Some of his patients travel for 12 hours by car to see him. If you are patient and persevering with the treatment, you will get better. Dr. Liebell and his family will treat you like the family you wish you had. I am so grateful for having met Dr. and Mrs. Liebell and Barbara." – Christine R., Virginia Beach, VA

Chapter 33

"Evidence-Based Medicine" Evil

Perhaps you have heard of the term, evidence-based medicine (EBM). This is popular medical jargon which, in my opinion is being inappropriately thrust upon doctors and patients as the new "gold standard" for medical care. What is evidence-based medicine? It is supposed to be the ultimate in scientific decision-making for doctors. Here's the problem: it seems to be incredibly unpopular with both doctors and patients! The concept of EBM opposes and violates numerous principles of many safe, effective, and time-tested treatment methods. What EBM suggests is that unless a health procedure has undergone gigantic and costly clinical medical trials, it is no good!

In my opinion, this proposed new standard for practicing medicine tragically reduces your humanity, panders to big business, and could potentially deprive people of their chance to receive safe, affordable, and effective treatment. So, let me shout it loudly and clearly that I do not currently represent the *Bio-energetic Individual Treatment Equation*© as evidence-based medicine. Technically, upper cervical chiropractic and auricular therapy qualify. However, I do not acknowledge the self-appointed gatekeepers of health care as capable or accurate in determining what constitutes effective treatment. I've got lots of patients who can do that quite fine. It is my suggestion to the public that doctors and patients join forces on a case-by-case basis, and determine what routes of evaluation and treatment to take. Logic, reason, and results should be utilized rather than rigid and financially-biased standards, which ultimately destroy people's opportunities to get well. Let us not forget that usage of FDA-approved drugs is considered "evidence-based medicine." Need I say anything more?

Any doctors who wish to criticize the *Bio-Energetic Individual Treatment Equation©* as not conforming to the standards of EBM may have at it. I could care less, and more importantly my patients won't flinch. I make no claims of anything other than overjoyed patients, who once believed they couldn't get well— now enjoying their lives as a result of extremely unconventional methods.

Whose Evidence is it Anyway?

Large clinical research trials cost up to tens of millions of dollars, and take years to accomplish. How many doctors who use inexpensive and drugless methods have the money to perform such a thing? Competency, compassion, skill, knowledge, patience, and some technology combine beautifully with the natural healing capacity of the human body. It trumps this pretentious evidence-based medicine without a doubt. It may be assumed by the public that statistics of success are what drive medical standards. In reality once again, it is more a matter of what has been subjected to very expensive and large-scale clinical research trials. And what methods get those done? Pharmaceuticals, of course! So, if you are expecting proof of success of the *Bio-Energetic Individual Treatment Equation©* with clinical research trials or evidence-based medicine, I must respectfully warn you that you will be disappointed. I do plan on conducting and publishing studies that will satisfy academic medicine's requirements too.

"It's just *anecdotal* evidence"

Individuals, groups, or factions whose mission it is to denigrate natural healing methods love to pontificate that results are based only on anecdotal evidence. The strict usage of the term refers to results that are not necessarily true or reliable because they are based on personal accounts rather than research. Yes, my patients and I offer anecdotal evidence. I cannot prove with

281

a costly clinical trial that my treatment helped them get well. For that matter, we cannot always prove they are well. We can only go by our bio-energetic testing standards and the patients' reports of how they feel and function. Keep in mind that many patients had no previous evidence-based medical proof of Lyme disease (and other illnesses or infections). They certainly had no proof of improvement. Otherwise they would never have sought my care in the first place. The majority of patients I see do not have CDC-approved positive Lyme disease blood tests. If there is no conventional medical proof of illness—the patient is not considered sick anyway! How can medical research be done if their tests and standards do not acknowledge the patients' illness?

History has shown that the people who have had the courage to shake up the establishment with new ideas have been the ones to produce scientific breakthroughs. Louis Pasteur, Albert Einstein, Linus Pauling, Samuel Hahnemann, and Paul Nogier are merely a few shining examples. None of their experiments would have conformed to the ridiculous standards of evidence-based medicine. They did indeed follow the scientific method. In my opinion, EBM is about statistics, conformity to convention, and money. It seems to have little to do with health and healing.

The *Bio-energetic Individual Treatment Equation's* components are derived from the work of scientists—people with credentials, credibility, results, and respect. We cannot suggest it as a treatment for Lyme, or any other disease of condition. It is a health care approach that has a different design for each person, and therefore will never conform to a standard treatment or protocol. It is simply bad medicine to automatically do the exact same thing to every patient who exhibits the same symptoms, injury or illness. Mainstream medicine rarely recognizes the person with the illness, but rather the illness itself.

I have never treated Lyme disease. I have successfully however, treated lots of *people* suffering the apparent chronic effects of tick-triggered illness. Scientific methods are those for which a result can be achieved by repeating the same process. It does not imply perfection, nor do my patients or I claim everybody gets well. Most do. They also understand that we are providing care, but making no claims of directly treating any disease in the conventional medical sense. All they care about is getting better. Safety and affordability to the best of my knowledge cannot be topped.

Each and every person is an individual, who responds in a unique matter to everything. I steer clear from Lyme wars and controversies by firmly acknowledging this fact as the core principles of the *Bio-Energetic Individual Treatment Equation.* © Holistic medicine is absolutely supported by science, despite what the gatekeepers of conventional medicine seem to aggressively dispute. Recognizing each person's individual needs, rather than generic protocols, drugs, therapies, and other treatments based on averages and statistics is critical. Treatments that are classified as alternative will ultimately become the scientific standards if the people demand them, and demonstrate that they will pursue them, despite health insurance companies' refusal to provide coverage. Parents have been paying for orthodontic braces out-of-pocket for many decades because they perceive the value of the medical service regardless of insurance coverage. I refer to my daughter, Darcy's $6,800 smile! I could help several victims of tick-triggered illness get well for that amount!

Doxycycline has been lauded as the cure for Lyme disease, and is portrayed as evidence-based medicine. I challenge those suffering from chronic tick-triggered illness to cast their votes. To date, there is little evidence that supports well-meaning and good-intentioned LLMD's prescription of potentially harmful long-term antibiotics. This equally does not invalidate any

283

positive results that have been achieved through such a practice. While I am obviously overall a critic of long-term antibiotics, it is not a matter of whether or not they are designated by the powers that be as evidence-based medicine.

Part Six:

Facing the New Frontier— What to Do Right Now!

"The high minded man must care more for the truth than for what people think." – Aristotle

Chapter 34

Spectators, Commentators, and Players—Why Some People Take Action and Get Well, While Others Stand On the Sidelines and Suffer

NOTHING is risk-free. LIFE is not risk-free. If you cannot accept risk, you are living on the wrong planet. What risk can you take which might alter the quality of life as you know it? Millions of people fall victim to the instant-gratification-society every year. The road to recovery is NOT quick and easy, nor does it come in a pill. Conventional medical care is the approach the *majority agrees with and accepts*. But sometimes what you *disagree* with the most can be the very thing you need. There are times when you must be careful of what you defend, protect, or reject. It just might be a life-changing gift in disguise.

Whenever I write an article, give a talk, or speak to an individual, I rejoice in the knowledge that some will act upon the information I give them, and go forth and get well. I also know that others are going to keep doing what they have been doing, no matter how poor the results. Trying anything new or different is out of the question. Their reason for not taking action is they do not believe it is necessary to _experience_ something to really understand what it is about. This kind of twisted logic might come from people who smoke and proclaim they understand they are risking lung cancer. Ask somebody terminally-ill if they truly understood the risks during their years of smoking. The answer would be, "no way!" There are some things that must be experienced firsthand to understand. A man can never truly understand what it feels like to have a baby… and somebody who has never suffered the effects of chronic tick-triggered illness can never understand what it is like to be a victim of it. Most importantly, only those who have experienced the transformation from sickness to health by applying the *Bio-energetic Individual Treatment Equation*© truly understand that the body can heal itself.

Spectators Don't Have a Clue What it is Like to be a Player!

Not knowing that something can be done often stops people from achieving many things in life. For over one hundred years it was believed that nobody could run a mile in under four minutes. No one really knew it could be done until a man named Roger Bannister *did it*. Out of nowhere, dozens of other people suddenly became able to do it too! That was because they <u>knew</u> it could be done. This same scenario has taken place with victims of chronic tick-triggered illness. The sick and suffering have been convinced that the human immune system is not capable of beating *Borrelia* bacteria. Some are convinced once one contracts Lyme disease—it is a life-sentence. Still more believe the only hope is long-term antibiotics and other risky, expensive, and complicated treatments. There was a time that I did not know we could conquer Lyme disease… until I saw my wife, Sheila, get it done! Subsequently dozens of other people did it right after her, from within the walls of my office… because *they* <u>knew</u> it could be done!

Overcoming the effects of chronic tick-triggered illness is absolutely achievable, because the human body has always been capable of doing so. There are people across America, whose bodies are naturally immune to Lyme *Borrelia* bacteria. They will tell you how they have been bitten by ticks their whole lives without suffering any problems. That is the whole point. It's the point so simple that hyper-educated minds can't grasp it. The solution has always been the <u>human immune system</u>. There is nothing far-fetched about this. Consider your workplace, school, church, or any group of people. There are <u>always</u> some people who don't get sick—when everybody else does. Whatever colds, flu, stomach viruses, or other germs are spreading around…they don't have a problem. Why? A well-functioning immune system. Plain and simple. It is the ultimate prevention. A powerful immune system has always been, and always will be the solution. This is the key to getting you started thinking bigger about your own immune system.

The secrets of the *Bio-energetic Individual Treatment Equation*© cannot be found in popular natural health websites or other books. That is because throughout my career I've been blessed to work with or study the "lost" works of several of the greatest doctors around the world. These were not celebrity physicians, known to the masses, but rather brilliant individuals who discovered and developed methods that produced magnificent results that did not conform to the *business* of medicine. Apply these approaches to yourself, as I show you, and I'm confident the results will delight you. I seldom use the word "always" when it comes to health care, as there are usually exceptions to any rule. Most patients who have applied the BITE have made magnificent improvements... not always all better… but usually *way* better.

Perhaps you are facing each day so physically and mentally challenged that you have no idea how you're going to make it through. Each morning when you wake up and think about what you could possibly do to get better, you want to go back to sleep. You loathe the idea of yet another treatment failing, yet you know that in your heart that you can't just give up, and this makes you even more anxious. You particularly dread the thought of getting your hopes up for another doctor's treatment. Will this treatment be more of the same thing? Will it drain my bank account like the others did? You wonder if the *road to health* could somehow be easier, and your future a lot more secure. More and more people are discovering every day that it can.

Imagine that such thoughts need never again shadow you like hounds in the night. Of course that does not mean that you will definitely get well. No method is perfect, and not everybody is capable of success. But it does mean that you have realistic hope based upon the results of others. Moreover, on those inevitable-but-rare occasions when a patient does not improve, there is little-to-no risk of *harm*. I challenge any critics or skeptics to find a treatment approach that can legitimately make that claim.

"I had always had complete faith in traditional medicine and doctors, but when you suffer from something for years and can't get any answers from traditional doctors, you start to look towards alternatives. Several years ago, I would have never even considered homeopathy [energy medicines] as a treatment, but now, I can't imagine my life without it. Knowing that there aren't any side effects and that in simple terms, it's just "reminding" your body to do what it's supposed to puts me at ease when putting something into my body. I feel amazing! Pretty much all of my symptoms have vanished and I now don't even remember what it was like being so sick. Dr. Liebell has turned my life around for the better and I feel back to my old self. I have a 3 month old baby boy, and if I hadn't received this treatment, I not only was healthy enough to get pregnant, but I also wasn't healthy enough to even consider taking care of a baby. He is the absolute joy of my life and I have to thank Dr. Liebell for getting me to the point where I can be the mother that I always dreamed of being."

- Erin J., Virginia Beach, VA
[Erin now has *two* beautiful and healthy children!]

Chapter 35

Your New Beginning: What to Do Right Now!

In life, if you want to arrive at a terrific destination, you must first have one. It all starts with a clear vision of what you want—something that really excites you. If your destination is an office with a physician eager and willing to prescribe you the latest drugs that will give you the temporary *illusion* that you are well, the *Bio-energetic Individual Treatment Equation©* is definitely not for you. If your destination is the office of a doctor who intends to cycle you on and off of *antibiotics...* you are barking up the wrong tree.

The truth is that we can never help the majority of people who need help the *most*. Why not? Because perhaps the majority of people will assume this health care approach is too good to be true. Even those who have spent obscene fortunes chasing Lyme disease without results may be too set in their ways with regards to conventional philosophy. For many, the unavoidable task is to first *unlearn* things they have to believe as Lyme disease treatment gospel. Our beliefs can move us forward or hold us back. If you believe you cannot be helped, even a little, you will never move forward. I have seen too many people NOT... and wilt away. But the vast majority of those who have tried have blossomed back like a flower that only needed water! I urge you to find out for yourself if you have a chance to blossom once again too.

"While visiting my friend, Nellie in Virginia, and making the discovery of that dreaded "bulls-eye" on her leg, and arm after her hiking the western mountains of Virginia, I honestly was at a loss as to where to turn to help her seek treatment. This friend of mine operates under a holistic approach to life and had been healthy enough to "hike the trails" for 5 days in her late 70s! Her condition was worsening, so, I turned to the internet to find an alternative to antibiotics which she was refusing to accept as her treatment (she was also doing her own research). I came upon Dr. Liebell's website, and, scheduled an appointment for her. The day she was to see the doctor her condition worsened to the point that one of her legs gave out. I had her hug a tree while I went for the car. The trip to the doctor's office seemed forever because I was so unsure what would happen next. She began treatment and several months later after experiencing many frightening hours and sleepless nights, she recovered. I wasn't about to leave her until I knew she was able to walk the street or the stairs without falling. Honestly, I have never seen such horrible symptoms (not even with cancer patients). I was not the patient, I was the witness (present nearly every hour) during the treatment. Dr. Liebell's treatment plan was affordable, and easier to follow than many "main-stream" practices. I thank Dr. Liebell and his staff for treating my friend, Nellie, and me, when we were in need of loving care. As with any illness, one has to believe you will get better, like you do with a common cold, and follow the advice of the doctor, when need be."

- Jill R., on behalf of Nellie H., Chesapeake, VA

My goal is to have it known throughout the Lyme disease community—today, in six months, in five years, in 10 years, and perhaps even in 30 years—that those using the *Bio-energetic Individual Treatment Equation©* consistently rank among the most extraordinary health recovery success stories in the world. Should you pursue it, I want to have you be recognized as someone who was intelligent enough to have realized conventional medicine's failure to fulfill its promise. Somebody who explored *other* approaches to overcome chronic tick-triggered illness. I want to see you recognized for inspiring well-founded confidence in a *natural* wellness-based system because you know what it did to help <u>you</u> finally get well. I will look forward to you sharing the privilege I have had—experiencing firsthand the mind-blowing power of the human immune system.

Comparative Costs and Safety

Money does matter. How it should be spent is up to the individual. I do believe that health should be everybody's highest priority. Anything that restores, improves, or maintains ones' health is a great investment. The Liebell family spends a considerable amount of money on the finest quality foods we can afford, as well as fitness equipment, pool memberships, and of course the bio-energetic products used in my practice. I have made some curious observations over the past twenty-three years in practice. One in particular is that people's willingness to pay to improve their health is not directly related to their wealth. I've seen rich people who balked at the notion of spending a couple of hundred dollars for an evaluation that could mean the difference between a life of misery versus health and happiness. In contrast, patients with low or even *no* income have been willing to do whatever necessary to pay for the care they needed.

Some folks maintain the attitude that if health insurance does not cover the costs of something, it must not be worth doing. I couldn't think of anything more peculiar than trusting insurance companies to make my health choices. There's another interesting thing about paying directly for a doctor's services versus having insurance pay for it. When people pay for the care out of their own pockets, they tend to be more committed to following instructions and getting results. When insurance pays for something, it seems like it is not as big of a deal. The financial risk seems to affect the attitude. In my opinion, the controversies of Lyme disease are ultimately money matters. Those who fight for Lyme disease awareness put great energy into trying to get long term antibiotic treatment endorsed and accepted by mainstream medicine. Why? Antibiotics are typically covered by most medical insurance! I view the outcry for allowing more antibiotics as pleading for costs to be covered—not a strong advocacy for them as a treatment. It seems logical because insurance companies routinely pay for antibiotics.

Why do you think people don't come to see me *first?* The conventional medical tests and at least some extent of antibiotic treatment are covered by health insurance. Insurance pays for initial doctor visits, blood tests, x-rays, MRIs, neurological tests, and medications with fees ranging from hundreds to tens of thousands of dollars.

The question is, would people seek out *those* tests and treatment as their first choice, if they had to pay for it?

Might they choose holistic medicine first? If we take insurance coverage out of the equation, conventional medicine is unaffordable to most people. Natural and holistic medicine is both affordable and effective.

The only real obstacle I have found for my patients has not been the costs of *my* care, but rather the burden suffered by the ghastly amounts of money already frittered away on previous unsuccessful care.

"I was experiencing debilitating headaches, vertigo, stomach paralysis, chronic fatigue, neck pain depression and anxiety from Lyme disease. I felt sick all the time and did not want to do or participate in anything. I had no strength to do anything and I had such bad anxiety and depression I could not function normally. I had been to family practitioners, gastric, liver, infectious disease, neurologists, endocrinologists, oncologists, cardiologists, sleep doctors and psychologists who prescribed numerous antibiotics, narcotics for pain, anti-fungal and anti-viral medicines as well as anti-depressants. I can honestly say that I have improved the most from using Dr. Liebell's treatment using chiropractic and homeopathic remedies. My painful headaches have been reduced. My stamina is improving so I can walk again. I have started to drive again since the vertigo is improving. I'm starting to get my life back again. My quality of life has improved immensely. I can do almost everything physically I was able to do before except that I am still working on getting my full strength back. I have been very impressed. Dr. Liebell knows how to listen and is very knowledgeable. If there is any doubt or question he will research and respond quickly! In this business timing is critical. Dr. Liebell has my complete trust when it comes to health and wellness issues. We both ask a lot of questions and do not accept the status quo. The energetic testing was pain free and very quick and easy. I didn't feel anything with the ear acupuncture treatment. If you don't believe that other than antibiotics could be a solution—you're missing out on a much better alternative. You feel so much better on homeopathic treatment and it works!"

- Anne M., Virginia Beach

I've treated countless since 1993 in my holistic health practice, and have observed some fascinating things. Invariably, those who rise to the top in both extent of improvement and ease of doing so, are those who possess (1) knowledge of the treatment methods being used, and (2) superior <u>dedication</u> to succeed. Both are absolutely necessary. If you are interested, we doctors trained in our BITE approach stand ready to provide you the knowledge, skills, and technology. But the dedication can come only from <u>you</u>. Are you motivated enough to invest, say, just a small fraction of what legions of victims of tick-triggered illness have been willing to invest in *their* health?

Here's what I mean... Counting all costs, the average patient has forked over $10,000-$80,000 (out-of-pocket) to other doctors, but report being no healthier than before...often worse! Yet every year, so many suffering souls stricken with the effects of tick-triggered illness seek out these doctors who claim expertise in health, yet appear, to my understanding to be willing to put people on antibiotics and other powerful drugs indefinitely. There is a Southwestern clinic that I'm told charges $30,000-$60,000 for 12-week rotating antibiotic protocols, which require treatment 5 days/week.

Many Internet forums and threads are inundated with bitter complaints about insurance coverage. It seems they believe that the solution to the effects of tick-borne illness is having medical insurance pay for long-term antibiotics. So it really comes down to dollars and cents. The question you have to ask yourself is, do you have as much motivation to get well as those who have been willing to pay such preposterous amounts of money for such treatment? Many of them watched a popular Lyme disease awareness documentary (and its sequel), and were convinced they needed long-term antibiotics, at all costs. Fortunately, the costs for BITE wellness treatment are nowhere near $80,000. It is laughable miniscule fraction of that, and it comes with a benefit that the antibiotic doctors could never dream of offering: the utmost of safety! You can wait for our government to fund research for holistic and natural healing methods. Perhaps someday wellness supplementation will be covered by insurance.

Please don't shoot the messenger, but holistic wellness care is not covered by insurance. You must be willing to make an investment in yourself that will pay dividends for the rest of your life. I make no apologies for the costs of my approach because compared to all others, the *Bio-energetic Individual Treatment Equation©* is a very *inexpensive* program. When one discovers something important enough, the goal is to make sure everyone who needs it can get it—not just the rich, entitled, or health-insured.

My mission—my grassroots effort is to become an unstoppable fighting force for victims of tick-triggered illness across the country, and confront the mysteries, while avoiding the wedge issues of Lyme disease involving antibiotics, politics, blood tests, and high-risk, and obscenely costly medical practices... and to get doctors across the country on board to train with us, so people don't have to come all the way to Virginia Beach to get well. If you are reading this book because you received it from a doctor I helped train in the BITE... congratulations to that doctor. He or she was brave and bold enough to fight convention and dare to be different—to help you get well.

Nobody has had to take out a second mortgage on their home to get well at the Liebell Clinic. Since 1993, I have a large and dedicated family of patients in my practice. However, I proudly report that it is a *small* family business. I have no need for a huge staff (with a payroll to go along with it). It's just my wife/office manager Sheila, our wonderful assistant Barbara, and me. My malpractice insurance costs a miniscule compared to antibiotic doctors because of the unparalleled *safety* of my methods. I do not require a legal fund to fight medical boards or patients suing for wrongful death, or abuse of prescription drugs.

The Liebell Clinic is a place that people are coming to, from around the country to get well. It is not one of those multi-million dollar imperial palaces, decked out with water fountains, granite countertops, original artwork, and other unnecessary

296

bells and whistles to influence you how good the doctor must be. None of those things help you get better. I lay out my own money for the development and production of the bio-energetic supplements my patients use. I do not make deals with, nor do I get kickbacks from drug companies. There are no pharmaceutical salespeople offering me free lunches and vacations to use their products.

The *Bio-energetic Individual Treatment Equation©* is unique. It is available to highly-motivated people, who are truly committed to getting well. On behalf of current and future BITE doctors, I invite you to join our elite circle of patients and friends. I also have a few requests for you to consider:

1) **You must be willing to share your experience with others in need.**

It would be living in fantasy land to expect this treatment system to ever become mainstream. The *business* of health care is predicated upon people being <u>sick</u>… not getting *well*. This is the harsh reality. Therefore, word-of-mouth is critical to the welfare of others who need help just like you. You will be exposed to evaluation and treatment methods available in only a few clinics in the entire world. But very few people will *believe* the results you would likely achieve. Therefore, I expect patients to tell others how they got well, and to refer others to clinics applying the *Bio-energetic Individual Treatment Equation.©*

2) **You must put any pre-conceived ideas you may have about treatment of Lyme disease aside.**

Other doctors, as well as nutritionists, herbalists, energy practitioners, etc. may have convinced you that it is necessary to do a great diversity of other things. Things like: gluten-free diets, liver cleanses, glutathione supplements, adrenal gland

297

supplements, chelation therapy, infrared saunas, dental filing removal, sun chlorella, and many others. Internet chat threads are loaded with Lyme sufferers exchanging advice on all kinds of things they are convinced you must do. If you are to succeed with the BITE, it is critical to clear your mind of what you've been taught in the past. The people who get the best and fastest results are the ones who resist the temptation to do MORE things. I promise you I am not being boastful or arrogant when I tell you the people who keep it simple—and follow the extremely easy and safe treatment (without causing more stress on their bodies with other things)… get the best results.

We want you to get well. We want it to be easy and simple. Many patients are so entrenched in Lyme culture and the ideas of LLMDs, nutritionists, herbalists, and other practitioners (and patients too) that they can't let go. I am politely suggesting to you that you will not help me or other BITE doctors to help you by trying to convince us of the necessity for these *other things*. Most doctors have professional access to nearly *any* herb, vitamin, antioxidant, cleanse or detoxification product on the market. We can obtain Rife machines, and just about any other gadget out there. But why waste *your* money on what does not work!

3) You must fully accept what true natural healing is, and what it is not.

Remember what I have said throughout this book about herbs, diets, and vitamin supplements. Everything obtained from nature does not serve to promote natural healing. There are all kinds of *poisonous* things from nature! True natural healing is when your BODY is the agent of cure… where it gradually and progressively improves its function and repairs and regenerates itself.

4) You must be willing to give up Lyme disease as your "identity."

Your problem is NOT Lyme disease, but rather a malfunctioning immune system, which has been unable to naturally manage all kinds of bacteria, viruses, fungi, larger parasites, chemicals, and other stresses. Obsessing over Lyme has been the downfall of many a poor soul. What a mess. Don't let this happen to you. If it has already, you've got to snap out of it—for your own good. It is the road to ruin. It is unrealistic and illogical to try treat each individual microbe by bombing them with drugs. Scientific evidence does not support that approach, as your body will not get stronger (quite the opposite). By applying the *Bio-energetic Individual Treatment Equation,*© we do NOT treat Lyme disease. We help PEOPLE whose immune systems are too dysfunctional to overcome a vast array of harmful microorganisms and other factors. Every symptom you suffer is NOT from Lyme disease *(you may not even have any medical proof of Lyme anyway—and that doesn't matter either).*

There you have it—the master secrets of recovery from tick-triggered illness. This natural health system is the result of many decades of research and development. I invite you to seize the moment, and give yourself the opportunity to be the next great success story, and stand apart from those who accept a life of misery, hooked on drugs, learning to cope with the pain, taking the word of so-called authorities—the naysayers, who put down anything naturally curative that isn't patented and profitable.

"The public needs to know my story! It is NOT another story of Lyme disease tragedy, hopelessness, and antibiotic controversy. My story is about triumph. Not just for myself, but many others. I hope it will help many more people get their lives back, just like I did.

I was a strong and healthy, athletic and energetic young woman. I played high school varsity softball, basketball, and volleyball, as well as college tennis. But by about age 40, with three little children, I was a train wreck. I struggled with fatigue, mood swings, joint pain, heart palpitations, and memory problems, among other symptoms. Driving my car, I'd forget where I was going. I felt like I was slowly dying inside. I would eventually discover Lyme disease to be the culprit. My husband is a wonderful chiropractor. He was the only one capable of doing anything to help me. But he knew it wasn't enough; something was missing. And he believed that my symptoms were real, even though tests didn't reveal anything, and no other doctors had any answers either. I thought I asked our family M.D. for a blood test for "West Nile virus." Except, because of my "brain fog," my voice said, "Lyme disease" instead! I never saw a tick or a bull's eye rash. Fortunately, the doctor was willing anyway. By sheer luck, it came back positive, which of course, is often not the case. This began my Lyme recovery odyssey.

We found out why I was miserable. But treatment attempts were even worse. Antibiotics were a colossal disaster. All they did was tear up my insides and make me feel worse. I tried many other treatments (conventional and "alternative"), but they all failed equally. Fortunately, my husband never gave up! He searched and searched for help—and help he finally found! To make a long story short, I fully recovered from chronic Lyme disease, and its related problems. But it wasn't some "miracle" herb, detoxification cleanse, nutritional program, or frequency machine. It most definitely was not from antibiotics.

I got well because of an extremely rare, but very sophisticated, holistic method, with origins from France and Germany. My husband found out about it while studying acupuncture with a doctor, who once had Lyme himself. The examination and treatment methods involved some very strange-sounding things. "Energy medicines" and acupuncture done just on the ear? It was hard to believe something so easy, safe, and simple could make such a difference. How could this help my body cure Lyme?

But it did. This method delivered me from of a lifetime of illness. It worked by helping g my own immune system to defeat the Lyme bacteria, viruses, fungi, and intestinal parasites. Slowly, but surely. Not in a day, or a month, but about one year. Every other method tries to kill the germs with chemicals taken from the outside! My own immune system eliminated the Lyme and all of the co-infections from the inside—without use of any medication whatsoever. It wasn't a direct treatment for Lyme disease—it strengthened ME, the PERSON poisoned by Lyme disease.

Once I was helped, my husband became expert in this natural method. He has been helping others get well ever since. It's so ahead of its time. It boggles the minds of so-called experts, who think drugs are the only answer. Too many people are suffering needlessly—not knowing that their own immune systems are capable of defeating Lyme disease. The CDC tells people that doxycycline will "cure" Lyme. Don't get me started! Doctors and documentaries are suggesting people need long-term antibiotics. But these doctors have no experience seeing what the human immune system is really capable of—with the right assistance. Victims of chronic Lyme disease travel from many states to see my husband, Dr. Donald Liebell. His patients, he, and I have the privilege of seeing people recover all the time now! But of course, few people will believe it. I was able to go back to work after 10 years of suffering. Why? Because the methods he uses to help others are what enabled me to be healthy enough to do so. It has been my mission and privilege to play a part. I spend hours on the phone with people, who need to know there is realistic hope—and that it has nothing to do with more antibiotics! Doctors don't have faith in the immune system's power, and neither do their patients. But I do. I am in awe of its healing power. I have had the privilege to experience it firsthand, and to see it in my husband's patients.

I do not apologize for screaming out to any Lyme disease sufferer who will listen, that they should seek care with my husband. Everybody deserves the same opportunity to get well that as I got. Dr. Donald Liebell helps chronic Lyme sufferers every day—whether or not any formal diagnosis confirms such a condition. And he does it without drugs! That is no small feat. Some might call it "miraculous." The so-called health authorities have let everybody down. Anybody that offers another way to solve a problem that doesn't involve pharmaceutical treatments has always been ridiculed. This attitude keeps people sick and getting sicker. Please give yourself a chance to get well just like I did, and no many, many more people from all over America.

Sheila Liebell, Virginia Beach

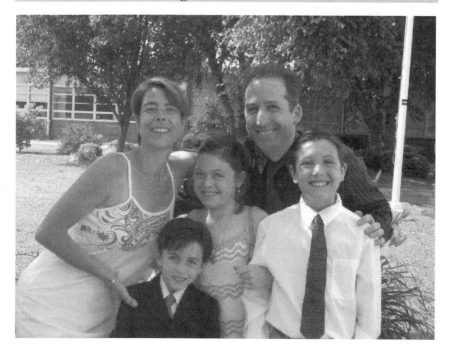

Chapter 36

Frequently Asked Questions

"Is it safe for me to take bio-energetic support supplements if I am also taking prescription, or over-the-counter medicines?"

YES, absolutely. They are are completely safe and compatible with any and all conventional medicines, and for that matter, any other treatments. There are NO drug interactions or side effects. The worst case scenario is treatment is ineffective.

"What about herbal remedies?

The same rules for pharmaceutical drugs apply for herbs, which like conventional drugs, are chemical in their effect.

"I'm taking antibiotics... can I apply the BITE?"

Yes. It is completely safe and compatible. I ethically do not discourage any patients from using any medical treatment. If you are *still* taking antibiotics, results will be much slower because one of the many significant side effects of long-term antibiotic usage is suppression of the immune system.

"Are bio-energetic supplements safe for children or pregnant women?"

I don't think there couldn't be a better choice of treatment for pregnant women. There are no side effects for the mother or developing baby. There is no chemical effect.

"Can I overdose with bio-energetic supplements?"

No. The concept of overdosing is not a concern. Treatments are not dosages in the conventional medical sense. Each spray delivers a single *exposure* of the beneficial frequencies—the informational imprints embedded in the product. One could drink the whole bottle with no danger; the body would take it as ONE exposure or dosage the same as one *spray!* It would only be a waste of money, but no harm to your body; there are no medicinal or pharmaceutical substances in any of the products. How OFTEN one takes the products is what matters. The bottom line is that one cannot overdose on something that is not a drug.

"Will it take a long time for me to get well with this approach?"

Your body certainly cannot eradicate a chronic illness or physical damage overnight. It is not a matter of how fast bio-energetic supplementation works… it's a matter of how your BODY works—and how complex your illness is. The treatment creates a triggering mechanism to support your body's healing on its own. Both injuries and chronic ill health take time to get better. This is life. A broken bone, properly treated, takes a solid three months to heal. If you're like most of my patients, you've tried many types of treatment for some time, with limited or no success. A chronic pain condition and/or illness may take years or even decades to develop. It is unreasonable to expect instant health from any true natural and holistic method. Most patients do notice at least some improvement within 6 months.

"Is this New Age Medicine? Could its usage compromise my religious principles?

I realize that there are various unusual methods in the alternative medicine field—some of which do have some principles contradictory to traditional faiths. You can rest assured that this is NOT the case with any of my treatment methods. There is absolutely no aspect of ANY Eastern mysticism, or anything at all that compromises anybody's religious principles.

"Is Homeopathic medicine endorsed by any trustworthy organizations?"

Homeopathy has been endorsed by the *World Health Organization, the Red Cross, the National Institutes of Health (NIH - USA), National Centre for Complementary & Alternative Medicine, (a U.S. Government agency) International Medical Volunteers Association.* Don't be fooled by the fact that the *American Medical Association* does not endorse it. Remember that it is a doctors' lobbyist organization that was formed largely to annihilate homeopathy in America. In Britain, France, The Netherlands, Norway, Germany, and Greece, homeopathy has been incorporated into their respective national healthcare systems. In Asia, especially India, government councils for the regulation and administration of homeopathy have been in effect for the last 75 years.

"What do I do if NEW symptoms or conditions arise while recovering from chronic old problems?"

Anybody can catch a cold, eat tainted food, or be exposed to any illness-causing factors. Or you can injure or stress your body in other ways. This means that even if you're progressively recovering from *chronic* illness or injury… you can develop NEW problems. This is certainly NOT a sign that your treatment is failing. You should additionally always consult with your local conventional physician for any appropriate evaluation. Bio-energetic testing and supplementation are NOT a replacement for your family medical doctor, other specialists, or their treatment. I do not represent this approach as diagnosis or treatment of any condition. It is complementary to conventional medical care. If you have an acute infection, medical emergency, or other situation (particularly those related to prescription medications), please contact your conventional medical doctor.

"What about AGE? Do younger people respond faster than middle aged or elderly patients?

It may seem odd, but age does not seem to play much of a role in effectiveness and speed of recovery. Some of my toughest cases have been teenagers, and some of the most extraordinary recoveries have been in patients in their seventies or eighties! Mainstream medicine, as well as the entertainment industry, and the media have the public convinced that age is much more significant than my patients' experience has shown it to be. Consider that a broken bone in a 5-year-old takes about 3 months to heal… as is the case for a 50-year-old. With proper treatment, healing time is not as much a function of age as might be thought. Physical DAMAGE to one's body is much more significant than age. A younger person may require much more time and bodily effort to repair and regenerate depending on the complexity and extent of illness and/or injury.

"How do I locate a clinic trained in applying the Bio-energetic Individual Treatment Equation (BITE)?"

To my knowledge, at the time of publishing this book there are two fully-functional clinics in North America:

The Liebell Clinic: Chronic Pain and Wellness Solutions: Dr. Donald Liebell, D.C.

477 Viking Drive Suite 170 Virginia Beach, VA 23452
(757) 631-9799 www.Hope4Lyme.com
Email: necksecret@gmail.com

Alternative Medicine Center—Nader Soliman, M.D.
14955 Shady Grove Road Suite 250 Rockville, MD. 20850
(301) 251-2335 Email: MyAlternatives@yahoo.com

More BITE practitioners are needed! All types of doctors and acupuncturists, who are interested in training should contact me at necksecret@gmail.com. Prospective patients may email me to see if there are other trained practitioners currently available.

Index

A

Acupuncture, 21, 96-99, 124, 128, 145, 151-179, 209, 213, 223, 237, 245, 253, 294, 301
Addison's disease, 67
adrenal glands, 53-54, 65-69, 203
AIDS, 62, 135-136, 199
ALS, 40, 76-77
Alzheimer's disease, 52
American Institute of Homeopathy, 189
American Medical Association (AMA), 126-127, 167, 190, 222, 247, 268-269, 305
Amygdala, 177
anecdotal evidence, 281-282
Anthrax, 71
Antibiotics
    antibiotic resistance, 71, 87,
    bacterial genocide, 10, 73
    blood-brain-barrier, 81, 113
    bull's eye rash, 16, 27, 76-77, 180, 300
    causing leaky gut, 105-112
    causing lowering of glutathione levels, 104
    direct treatment of Lyme disease, 180
    effect on protozoan parasites, 65
    effect on viruses, 50, 57-58, 194, 257
    effectiveness, 20, 22, 76, 90,
    end of era, 3, 12
    fibromyalgia, 37
    fungal consequences, 58-61
    herbs, 114-115
    Herxheimer reactions, 100-103, 244
    indefinite courses, 4, 12, 43, 95
    insurance coverage, 45, 230, 293
    malpractice insurance, 296
    misuse and abuse, 10, 60, 73, 86, 110
    probiotics, 107-111
    questioning as cure, 44, 78-80, 88, 120, 211, 263, 271, 283
    rise of gluten intolerance, 110
    side effects, 3, 10

silver bullet, 147
statistics, 29
suppression of immune system, 303
suspected Lyme disease, 43
treatment battlefield, 23
wedge issue, 5, 296
Why Antibiotics are Not the Answer, 56, 71-88
antibiotic-resistant bacteria, 3, 11, 72, 86-87
antibodies, 106, 133, 139
antidepressant drugs, 36, 67, 85, 85, 95, 185
antigen, 133
anti-inflammatory drugs, xi, 86, 107, 112, 250
antioxidants, 23
Arboviruses, 49
Aristotle, 117, 286
Aspergillus, 59
Atlas Orthogonal, 227-229
Audio books, 98
Auricular Bio-energetic Testing (ABT), 97, 159, 161, 162, 166, 167, 171-175
auricular therapy, 96- 100, 121, 151-179, 181, 196, 209, 219, 223, 245, 252, 253, 280,
autoimmune, 38-39, 57, 62, 83, 105, 128, 137, 230

B

Big Pharma, 148, 190
Babesia, 62, 81, 108
Bannister, Roger, 287
Bartonella, 81, 83
Battlefield Acupuncture, 156
battlefields, 22-25, 91
Bell's palsy, 41, 194
bio-electric fields, 142-167, 190
Bio-energetic Individual Treatment Equation (BITE)
    antibiotic resistance, 72-73
    clearing energetic blockages, 97, 173-181, 219
    comparative costs and safety, 292-296
    conventional medicine, 75, 119, 148, 158, 176, 201. 261, 265, 266, 283, 291, 293, 303
    detoxification systems, 25
    evidence-based medicine, 280-284

glutathione, 3, 103-104, 297

immune system, 122, 129-141

improving physiology, 181

internal wisdom of the body, 84

metal chelation, 54-55

pain management and rehabilitation, 181, 241, 279

safety, 85, 119, 189

sleep, 93-99

whole foods, 69, 96, 104. 110, 111, 238-240

blood-brain-barrier, 81, 113

Biofilm, 82

bipolar disorder, 62

Blaser Martin J., 86-87

Blastocystis hominis, 62

blockages of energy, 66, 97-98, 141, 173-178, 219, 255

blood tests, 2, 5, 12, 27, 28, 29, 39, 43, 45, 50, 143, 157, 159, 170, 211, 250, 282, 293, 296,

Bogduk, Nikolai, 231

Borrelia, 1, 4, 11, 13, 21, 23, 27-83, 109, 129, 135, 137, 140, 164, 180, 181, 194, 211, 217, 218, 230, 277, 287

Bourdiol, Rene, 177

brain fog, 47, 49, 50, 176, 300,

bugs (also see arthropods), 61, 277

bull's eye rash, 9, 16, 27-29, 76, 157, 180, 300,

Burr, Harold, 144-159, 171

business of medicine, 43, 268, 288

C

cadmium toxicity, 53-54, 82

caffeine, 66, 96

cancer, 51, 57, 59, 86, 100, 104, 118, 136, 138-140, 144, 149, 168-170, 183, 232, 236-239, 242, 286,

Candida (yeast infection), 54, 58, 72, 80, 136

cat's claw, 81, 113

cats, (also see *Toxoplasma*), 63

CD57, 133

Centers for Disease Control (CDC), 20, 27-28, 57, 63-64, 71-72, 76, 82, 87, 267, 282,

cervical spine (neck), 224, 226-234,

Chabris, Christopher (*The Invisible Gorilla*), 158-159

chelation therapy, 54, 298

chicken pox, 135
chiropractic, 169, 221-234
chronic fatigue syndrome, 36, 37, 40, 57, 195
 chronic vs. acute illness, 31-33, 46-51, 128, 155, 217
cigarette smoke, 52-53, 240
Cinchona bark, 186
cingulate gyrus, 177-178
circadian rhythm, 93, 97,
cleanses, 3, 17, 64, 83, 90, 264, 297
Clostridium difficile, 71
Coccidiomycosis, 59
Coffee, 65-66, 187
cognitive dysfunction, 39, 41, 68, 177, 278
coherent energy transduction, 197
co-infections, 30, 35, 109, 211
colds, 43, 52, 56, 57, 137, 202, 211, 243, 278, 288,
complementary medicine, v, x, 156, 183, 248, 254-255, 305
Consumer Reports, 238
copper toxicity, 54, 67, 82
corpus callosum, 175-176
costs of care, 3, 35, 54, 60, 73, 121, 292-296
Coxsackie virus, 50
Cryptococcus, 49, 59
Cryptosporidium, 62, 108
Cyberchondria, 33
Cysteine, 103

D

dementia, 52
dental fillings, 3, 53, 54
depression, 36, 41, 47, 52-54, 67, 95, 141, 177, 185, 210, 294,
detoxification, 24, 25, 51-55, 83, 89-103, 115, 116, 127, 129, 178, 203, 298, 300,
diagnosis, 1, 2, 8, 9, 11, 20, 22, 23, 26-88, 90, 100, 106, 108, 112, 125, 126, 129, 139, 157, 163-164, 168-169, 175-176, 181, 185, 195, 196, 211, 218, 226, 253, 254-259, 275, 305,
diarrhea, 41, 80, 187
diet, 5, 16, 51, 69, 87, 110, 111, 125, 127, 129, 180, 186, 216, 223, 235-240 , 255, 258, 264, 297-298
dizziness, 47, 50, 53, 75, 104, 163, 164, 191, 209, 212,

DNA, 46, 51, 78, 114, 145, 199, 200, 206,
documentary film, 169, 200, 278, 295
double-blind research study, 140, 254
Doxycycline, 41, 45, 79, 80, 82, 83, 119, 120, 263, 271, 283, 301,

E

ear acupuncture (see auricular therapy)
Ehrlichia, 81
Einstein, Albert, 31, 117, 118, 142, 235, 282,
electro-dermal screening, 145
Electroencephalogram (EEG), 46, 144
electromagnetic fields, 66, 159-166
ELISA, 45
Emotions, 66-67, 177
Encephalitis, 46-50, 57, 59
Entamoeba histolytica, 62
Enteroviruses, 49
Epstein-Barr virus (EBV), 48, 53, 57, 195
erythema migrans, 27 (see bull's eye rash)
evidence-based medicine, 280-284
exercise, 24, 66, 104, 125, 127, 142, 180, 192, 220, 223, 227, 240, 258, 272,

F

fatigue, 16, 21, 30, 32, 35, 37, 40, 41, 48, 52-54, 57, 65-69, 90, 104, 106, 109, 141, 163, 191, 195, 243, 260, 300,
FDA, 231-232, 263, 279, 311
fibromyalgia, 9, 30, 43, 44, 108, 163, 195, 209, 218, 226-227
Flexner Report, 148, 190
Fluoride, 96
food allergies, 72, 75, 86, 105, 110
free radicals, 103
functional medicine, 114, 126-128
fungus/fungi, 35, 38, 41, 49, 57-64, 72, 83, 100, 111, 132, 133, 136, 138, 243, 278-279, 299, 301,
G

Galileo, 161
Gastrointestinal, 52, 86, 106, 110, 191, 210, 217

Genetics, 7, 33, 40, 47, 51, 66, 91, 104, 128, 134, 149, 216, 218, 229, 230, 240, 258,
Giardia lambia, 62, 108-109
Glutamine, 103
Glutathione, 3, 103-104, 297
Gluten, 75, 106, 110, 297
Glycine, 103
Gonzalez, Nicholas, 232
gut bacteria, 90, 111, 124,

H

Hahnemann, Samuel, 56, 183, 186, 282,
hair loss, 53
headaches, 36, 41, 47-50, 52, 63, 106, 141, 163, 164, 188, 191, 213, 214, 230-232, 249, 278, 294,
healing crisis, 241, 244
Health care system, 7, 11, 21, 31-33, 37, 189
Heartburn, 52, 83
Helicobacter pylori, 100, 168
helminth parasites, 41, 61, 62, 64
herbs, 2, 3, 5, 13, 16, 17, 23, 54, 74, 81-83, 90, 113-117, 127, 129, 166, 184, 188, 189, 194, 205, 206, 238, 245, 251, 256, 258, 264, 279, 297, 298, 300, 303,
herpes viruses, 48, 62
Herxheimer reactions, 13, 100-102, 244
Hippocampus, 177-178
Hippocrates, 16, 183-187, 219
HIV, 135-136, 147, 199
Hodgkin's disease, 140
holistic dentists, 53
Homeodynamics, 252,
Homeopathic Pharmacopeia of the United States, 193
Homeopathy, 55, 75, 80, 82, 91, 96, 97, 124, 126, 141, 151, 153, 155, 161, 164, 166, 169, 178, 182-193, 199, 201, 209, 213, 219, 222, 223, 238, 244, 245, 247, 249, 252, 260, 262, 265, 289, 294, 304, 305
Hormones, 51, 65, 94-96, 144, 162, 235
human cells, 56, 61, 67, 78, 133, 138
Human Microbiome Program, 86

I

Iceman, 26
IDSA, 20
ILADS, 20
Immune system, Chapter 18 (and throughout entire book)
informational imprints, 196-206, 303
injuries and damage, 33, 118, 128, 144, 155, 162, 216, 226, 276-277, 279, 282, 304-305
innate immunity, 134
insects, 41, 49, 57, 61, 138, 249
Internet, 8-9, 33-34, 80-81, 87, 106, 129, 179, 291, 295, 298,
invisible gorilla experiment, 158-159

J

Josephson, Brian, 201
Journal of Whiplash and Related Disorders, 201, 226

K

Kerr, Patrick, 230
Klebsiella pneumonia, 71

L

Lyme literate Medical Doctor (LLMD), 3, 4, 21, 74, 104, 120, 283, 298
Law of Similars, 185
Lead, 52, 82
leaky gut, 105-112
learning disabilities, 52
L-fields, 144-147, 159
Liebell Clinic, 23, 111, 179, 215, 234, 250-251, 264, 296, 306
light filters, 160
Lou Gehrig's disease (see ALS), 39
Lupus, 38, 44
lymphatic system, 59, 90, 139-140

M

macro-parasites, 41, 49, 61-62
Maslow, Abraham, 85
Mayo Clinic, 59

mechanical problems, 220

melatonin, 93-99, 176

memory loss, 16, 41, 47, 52, 53, 79, 82, 106, 133, 148, 177, 178, 191, 210, 212, 213, 300,

meninges, 47, 228

mental illness, 7, 18, 33, 46, 50, 62, 79

mercury, 51, 53, 82, 186

metal toxicity, 51-55, 178, 203,

methyl-tetrahydrofolate reductase (MTHFR), 91

microorganisms, 8, 35, 37, 40, 56, 62, 67, 78-79, 83, 89, 96, 129, 133, 134, 219, 273, 278, 299,

micro-parasites, 41, 49, 61

Migraines, 36-37, 43, 53, 163, 194, 212, 213, 218

mimicking illnesses, 36-40, 106, 219

Missing Microbes (Blaser), 86-87

molds and mildews, 39, 55, 57, 269, 277,

monocytes, 139

mononucleosis, 57, 191, 195

Montagnier, Luc, 199, 200, 206

Morgellons disease, 50

MRI, 39, 46, 50, 144, 157, 163, 170, 175, 209, 250, 273, 293,

MRSA, 11, 71

Multiple Sclerosis, 38-40, 54, 194, 218, 230-231

Mycotoxins, 39, 59

N

National Center for Complementary and Alternative Medicine (NCCAM), 156, 183

National Institutes of Health (NIH), 27, 63, 74, 82, 121, 149, 305,

nervous system, 39, 49, 51, 59, 65, 79, 144, 159, 163, 187, 219, 221, 232

neuro-electric therapy, 97, 174, 178

Newton, Isaac, 142, 217

Niemtzow, Richard, 156

Nogier pulse reflex, 160-161, 171

Nogier, Paul, 153, 154, 159-162, 171-172, 174, 177, 179, 282

Norovirus, 549

NOVA, 26, 169

O

Obsession with Lyme, 29, 49, 57, 67, 71, 82, 103, 107, 109, 159, 299

Ockham, William of, 117
opioid drugs, 83
Oschman, James, 143, 200
Osteopaths, 126, 179, 256
Oz, Mehmet, 143

P

Painkillers, 77, 85-86, 214, 250
Paracelsus, 27, 131, 182-182
parasites (see micro-parasites, macro-parasites, protozoan parasites)
Parkinson's disease, 40, 52, 231
Pasteur, Louis, 40, 271, 282
Pathogens, 24, 37, 56, 74, 113, 132, 136-138, 203
Pediatric Autoimmune Neuropsychiatric Disorders Associated with Streptococcal Infections (PANDAS), 62
perceptual blindness, 158
peripheral neuropathy, 30, 36, 37, 43, 194, 218
PICC lines, 74
pineal gland, 94-99, 176
placebo effect, 121-123, 252, 261-274
Plasmodium falciparum, 62
pneumonia, 71, 83, 212
post-traumatic stress disorder (PTSD), 177
post-treatment Lyme disease syndrome (PTLDS), 41, 180, 218, 221, 263
POTS disease, 194
Pregnancy, 63, 66, 80, 119, 191, 214, 289, 303
primary vs. secondary conditions, 48, 217-226, 255
probiotic supplements, 58, 79, 107, 110-111
protozoa, 35, 41, 46, 49, 61-64, 110
psychiatric disorders, 18, 36, 46-50, 62, 74, 104, 109, 157, 210, 251

Q

quackery, 261-271

R

rebounding exercise, 140
reflux, 52, 83
resonance, 144, 161-168
reticular formation, 150, 155
Rife machines, 14, 100-102, 129, 264-264, 298

Rockefeller John D., 148, 190
Royal Family of England, 183
R-zone, 177

S

salads and parasites, 63
Salmonella, 136
Samento, 81, 113
Saunas, 298
Schopenhauer, 125
seasonal affective disorder (SAD), 95
seizures, 47, 63, 249
self-diagnosis, 33, 275
self-healing vs. self-correcting, 220
Shingles, 48, 135
Simons, Daniel, 158
sinus infections/sinusitis, 59-60, 245
size of bacteria viruses and human cells, 78
sleep cycle, 93-99, 128, 235
Smithsonian Magazine, 79
Soliman, Nader, x-xii, 155, 161, 172, 175, 177, 179, 186, 252, 306,
Sperry, Roger, 233
Spine, 35, 154, 219, 220-234, 264
spirochaete bacteria, 39, 62, 79
spleen, 133, 140
streptococcus, 62, 120
stress, 65-68, 96, 101, 105, 107, 110, 117, 127, 135, 137, 159, 160, 177, 205, 216, 218, 239, 240, 243, 251, 275, 298, 299, 305
sunlight, 80, 235
superbugs, 71-72, 135
Sweat Roy W., 227
Szent-Gyorgyi, Albert, 180

T

T-cells, 133
Tesla, Nikola, 142, 173
thalidomide, 119
thymus gland, 133, 140
tick bite, 27-28, 39, 41, 108, 137, 202, 217, 230,
Tourette syndrome, 62

toxins, 24, 39, 50, 54-57, 59, 65, 83, 89-92, 100-102, 106, 117, 127, 136-137, 162, 164, 192, 219, 242-244,

Toxoplasma gondii, 62-64, 81

traditional Chinese medicine (TCM), 152, 160, 173,

Treponema pallidum, 62, 79

Trypanosoma cruzi, 62

Tufts University, 149

Typhoid Mary, 136

U

upper cervical care, 224-234

V

Vaccination, 134

Varicella zoster, 48, 135

Vegetables, 59, 63, 96, 111, 238, 259

Vioxx, 123, 248

Virchow, Rudolf, 71

Virginia's Lyme Task Force, 29

viruses, 16-17, 34-41, 46-57, 61, 62, 64, 72, 78, 100, 132-138, 195, 199-202, 243, 259, 277-279, 288, 299-301,

vitamin B6, 96

vitamin C, 17, 104

vitamin D, 104, 170, 235-237

Voll, Reinhold, 145

W

Walnuts, 64, 96

water memory, 199-206

weak links, 217-219

Western Blot, 9, 28, 35, 45, 157, 180

white blood cells (leukocytes), 133-134, 138-140

Williams, Montel, 230-231

World Health Organization, 155, 305

worms (helminths), 35, 41, 49, 58, 61-62, 83, 108, 138

wormwood, 64

Y

Yale University, 143-144, 147, 149, 157

yeast (see *Candida*)

317

Made in the USA
Middletown, DE
22 October 2021